MW00978498

Creating Hospitals
We Can Trust

Creating Hospitals We Can Trust

Jane Lloyd

Writers Club Press
San Jose New York Lincoln Shanghai

Creating Hospitals We Can Trust

All Rights Reserved © 2002 by Jane Adams Lloyd

No part of this book may be reproduced or transmitted in any form or by any means, graphic, electronic, or mechanical, including photocopying, recording, taping, or by any information storage retrieval system, without the permission in writing from the publisher.

Writers Club Press
an imprint of iUniverse, Inc.

For information address:
iUniverse, Inc.
5220 S. 16th St., Suite 200
Lincoln, NE 68512
www.iuniverse.com

ISBN: 0-595-21883-0

Printed in the United States of America

To my talented sister

Nancy

CONTENTS

Acknowledgments

I am most grateful to my husband Robert for his unwavering support throughout the writing of this book. His patience and total acceptance of my commitment allowed me the time and freedom so essential for such a project.

Each of the other members of my family provided their own unique support. My daughter Melanie, in addition to her belief in me and her consistent encouragement, gave much of her time and assistance and contributed considerably to the quality of the writing. Her suggestions about style and her take-no-prisoners approach to the editing enabled me to maintain a professional tone yet at the same time "tell it like it is," which I was so determined to do. My son Dwight, his wife Chanda, and my grandchildren provided the love and encouragement that makes such a difference when one embarks on an arduous and uncertain journey. And my sister, Pat Torbert, also a nurse, provided both a sister's love and enthusiasm as well as her own contribution to the content of the book.

Others have offered both support and practical assistance. My childhood companion, nursing school roommate and lifelong best friend, Pat Tindal, provided valuable input from her career in obstetric nursing. She is one of the primary sources for Chapter III. Saundra Stewart, an experienced Intensive Coronary Care Unit nurse and manager, for whom I have had enormous respect both as a friend and a colleague over the years, was also an important resource. Without the assistance of friends like Margie Swartout and Jim Tindal, I would have had a much more difficult time acquiring those proficiencies that are essential to writing today. Both Margie and Jim possess that natural talent and patience so welcome (and often illusive) in teachers of computer skills.

Finally, I have had the honor, over the years, of working with many excellent health professionals, managers and executives. Without my associations with such knowledgeable and dedicated persons, and without both the input and inspiration of one former executive in particular, this book could never have had the substance and breadth necessary to confront such an issue.

FOREWORD

Years ago, when corporations first began buying hospitals in a few lucrative communities, they were touted as good business managers who would save us money and make the profits necessary for growth. This was music to the ears of the leaders of community hospitals who usually operated in the red. Physicians, nurses and other health professionals were happy as corporate money flowed in for equipment and expansion. Thus began a revolution, both insidious and tumultuous, that not only changed our community hospitals but also changed the course of almost all other facets of the health care business.

As corporations gained a foothold in hospital care, a far-reaching dark side of the revolution began to unfold. Many of the management strategies correlated precariously with patient welfare. Some were directly harmful. With focus on finance and ignorance of the professional processes that facilitate healing, CEO's soon began cutting back on professional staff at the bedside and reducing the patient's length of stay. Emergency rooms shifted indigent patients to other facilities. Deals with pharmaceutical companies and other suppliers intruded into physicians' treatment decisions. Continuing education for professional staff decreased, and hospital managers began an aggressive campaign of indoctrinating the previously inattentive doctors, nurses and other health professionals on the sanctity of budget. Everyone developed the art of meeting the reimbursement criteria of Medicare and the private insurer, and collectors pursued patients and families who were slow to pay their out-of-pocket share of hospital costs.

Designing our hospitals to Wall Street specifications, relegating the sick and injured to market share, resulted in more than dishonor to the mission of hospitals. It also set into motion today's out-of-control cost spiral throughout the entire health care industry.

A backlash from various predictable sources against the increasingly profitable hospital corporations was the first indicator of redirection and spread of the revolution. Amid the extraordinary wealth amassed by a few corporate executives as well as extravagant salaries, bonuses and other benefits to droves of lesser executives, both the government and the private insurance industry began making changes in their criteria for reimbursement. Other healthcare-related industries began to increase their own profit margin. Many community-owned hospitals, quick to distinguish themselves as "not-for-profit," also became more competitive by forming alliances and adopting some of the corporations' tactics.

Today, some of the practices of the past are more moderate. Yet, costs continue to rise, and the sale of health care resembles far too closely that of a non-essential service. In the tradition of discount shopping chains, an abundance of minimally trained workers take care of "customers" while an abundance of managers, consultants, and marketing experts take care of business. If individual hospital CEO's do not make their hospitals profitable enough, higher-level executives will find someone who can. Thus, CEO's often take the seemingly least risky, most immediately beneficial route of cutting costs at the level of service, although they may wish to do otherwise.

Meanwhile, physicians and nurses, in conflict with their professional imperatives, find themselves in complicity with a system that compromises their practice and extinguishes their spirit. Legislators find the system too complicated to approach. News media miss the right questions. And now the public, more from a sense of powerlessness than apathy, accepts hospital care as just another business enterprise, albeit one that holds considerable power over their lives. We have an odd relationship with our community hospital that is at once both adversarial and fiduciary. None of this is what we want; yet, it is the path we are taking together.

As always, there is a less-traveled road. It is accessible to those who have a clear vision, an explicit sense of direction, specific strategy and the resolve to stay the course. We can create hospitals, corporate or otherwise, that will serve their patients well and at the same time retain the necessary profitability for growth and modernization. This is today's task for executives, professionals, legislators and community leaders with integrity and courage.

INTRODUCTION

This book is for anyone interested in promoting, providing or receiving good hospital care. Its purpose is to assist readers in both identifying and helping to create trustworthy hospitals instead of the unsafe, assembly line businesses in which we all too often find ourselves or our loved ones. It is for the patient, family member and health professional at the bedside as well as the executive who must maintain the institution's financial integrity and profitability while creating the environment in which professionals can do their best work.

Although it focuses on the practice of nurses and physicians and on the hospital management by CEO's, all of whom are vital to resolving problems, it primarily addresses the public. Just as public education is not merely an issue for teachers, the quality of hospital care is not only an issue for health professionals and executives. Because virtually all of us will need a hospital at some time, often during major life events, hospital quality is a major public concern. For those with chronic illnesses, frequent hospitalization can become a way of life. Therefore, it is we the people who must be a driving force in reform. Among us are journalists, so necessary to an informed society, and legislators who seek insight into an unfamiliar domain.

I would not presume to address all health care issues, or even all hospital issues. Such an undertaking is beyond my scope and that of anyone else. One of the major obstacles to effecting solutions to the problems of our health care system is the fact that the issues are so numerous they become overwhelming. Would-be problem solvers with sweeping proposals often end up accomplishing little. Therefore, this book narrows its focus to the quality of hospital care, that is, the direct care rendered by nurses and physicians at the bedside of hospitalized patients.

Naturally, many issues are interrelated. The quality of direct patient care that is or is not possible in hospitals relates both directly and indirectly to costs. Quality determines the incidence of avoidable complications, revolving-door hospitalizations and lawsuits — all extremely expensive propositions. Quality directly correlates with mortality rates. And quality in working conditions is the greatest determinant of the abundance or dearth of practicing nurses.

A positive development in recent years is that the public has begun accepting more responsibility for personal health as well as taking a more authoritative approach when dealing with hospitals. Regular exercise, healthy diet, vitamin supplementation and adequate sleep are frequent subject matter for popular television shows and magazine articles. Physical exams include an increasing array of routine screening procedures, whether indicated by symptoms or not. Today's well-informed patients have long been seeking second opinions, and when hospitalization is necessary, they may arrive with any one of the take-charge-of-your-hospital-stay books under their arm.

The gradual rise of such preventive and empowering measures is without question one of the most important advances in "medicine" of our time. Yet, as important as these things are, they may make no difference whatsoever when one becomes a patient in a hospital. As patients, we may not always find it possible to keep a watchful eye on hospital workers or to stand up for ourselves at every turn. We may not be able to verify the credentials of the person at our bedside or observe if caregivers wash their hands. We may not be able to discuss with the doctor or nurse the appropriateness of one course of treatment over another. Such precautions are not likely if we have been transported bleeding or in shock from an accident scene. The same can be true if for any reason we are unable to communicate or if we are disoriented or, for that matter, just sick.

Some say that if we are hospitalized we should have a family member with us around the clock to insure our safety and good care. That is a sad commentary on the perception of hospitals, but more than that, heeding such advice does *not* assure our safety and good care. In the first place, family members will not be present during many procedures or in certain areas such as ICU's, operating rooms, recovery rooms, cardiac cath labs, nurseries and many others. They are likely to leave the bedside during an emergency in deference to hospital personnel and others who are giving aid to their loved one. Even when family members are present, their vigilance and input by no means insure the best medical decisions or nursing processes.

Even the well-informed cannot always be expected to participate rationally in medical decision-making affecting family members. Twenty years ago, I waited with my family outside the Intensive Care Unit where my brother lay dying. A young resident came to us often to keep us informed even when there was little to say. With great compassion, he told us several times during the course of three days that my brother would not survive and that the time was near. We listened intently, hanging on the doctor's every word, as families do in this kind of situation. But we could not hear him. We were incapable of assimilating such information, and we continued to discuss what the best possible medical decisions should be. The resident quietly waited, nodded, allowing us to go on, even though he knew that nothing we were going to do would change the outcome. He understood that a sudden catastrophic event had left our family unable to comprehend what was before us.

Naturally, there is no question that the presence of family members can make an important difference. Their love and support alone may sometimes determine the outcomes for patients because caring for the spirit is important to healing the body. Obviously, it is also beneficial to have an advocate. But hospitalization generally involves stress, and stress may render family members less capable of thinking as clearly as they normally would, even if they possess the necessary specialized knowledge, which they usually do not.

Patients and family members know if information from professionals does or does not sound logical to them, and they know when they are or are not treated with kindness and respect, but that is often all they know. Regardless of their intellectual or educational level, they have no sure way of recognizing when they are, or are not, getting appropriate care, and they often do not judge their care realistically.

Sometimes, upon being discharged from the hospital, grateful (and relieved) patients and families thank the staff profusely or fill out hospital care evaluation forms with high marks. Based on their knowledge, they perceived their care to be what was reasonably expected, the staff was accommodating, and everyone was nice to them. But niceness is not the measure of quality. Furthermore, because a significant portion of service takes place outside the presence of the patient and family, they can easily be unaware that the complication they developed was avoidable, that mistakes occurred, or the staff omitted important aspects of care.

Almost all patients and families are inclined to be cooperative with the hospital staff; extremely few are adversarial from the start. They naturally want to establish and maintain a good relationship with those who will be involved in their healing. They want to interact knowledgeably in what is, to them, an uncertain situation and unfamiliar environment. Most patients are more than willing to do their part so that physicians, nurses and other health professionals can make the best decisions and render the best care.

Even so, despite phenomenal advances in diagnostic and treatment technology, patients are not confident that their care will be competent and mistake-free. Their hospital may be controlled, not by their own community, but by a distant enterprise for which the first priority is a profitable bottom line. Assembly-line care, often rendered by cheaply-hired non-professionals, may place their safety and dignity at risk. They know that cost-cutting and the resulting decline in hospital service is taking a toll in increased patient complications and mortality rates, that patients sometimes receive the wrong medications, develop hospital-acquired infections and return home worse than they were before. They hear news reports that medical mistakes cause tens of thousands of deaths per year.

All of this constitutes a troubling situation that many individuals feel unable to challenge. Since boycott is not an option, the only alternative patients and families have is through the lawsuits they are now seeking in unprecedented numbers, though far less often than they justifiably could.

But lawsuits are hardly solutions; they are too late, and they only raise our costs — enormously. We are still left with the knowledge that when we are hospitalized, even in the company of family, we will place our health and safety in the hands of others. We have no choice but to trust our hospitals, and that is true whether we are knowledgeable, ignorant, assertive, timid, wealthy or indigent. Regardless of whether our hospital is good or bad, once we become patients, trust them we must.

Whatever we do to insure that we have trustworthy hospitals must therefore be done before the fact. It is on that premise that this book seeks to support the public by revealing precisely what constitutes good quality care and how to recognize its presence or absence in any hospital. Readers will be able to determine easily whether their hospital has instituted the conditions that are most likely to insure safe, competent and professional care when they need it.

This book also addresses some of the difficulties facing physicians. They have watched the quality of patient care decline and felt their own professional integrity threatened. Amid their complaints of less time for patients, dwindling and inconsistent professional nursing staffs also afford them less substantive and productive working relationships with bedside caregivers. Financial incentives and other pressures to which doctors are subjected can negatively affect their patient-care decisions and go against the ethical grain of their profession. They have begun to find very tiresome the dictates of hospital managers and distant managed care executives who possess neither the credentials nor the facts to make physicians' individual medical-practice decisions. While physicians are legally responsible for their treatment decisions, HMO's make such decisions without consequences, though that may soon change.

Many physicians also feel that even teaching hospitals now have less commitment to education, increasing the amount of residents' routine work and decreasing their learning opportunities. The once-powerful American Medical Association has lost much of its clout to corporations, and for the first time, medical school enrollment is declining. Some of today's doctors are reluctantly looking at unions, though the idea is repugnant to them because the possibility of deliberately withholding services has devastating implications for professional ethics.

While this book does not directly address all of these issues, it makes clear that the hospital service patients receive profoundly affects the quality of medical diagnosis and treatment. This will seem a foregone conclusion to many physicians, even those who do not fully understand the elements that comprise good hospital care systems, but it eludes the notice and understanding of other physicians. Consequently, they may freely offer ill-informed recommendations for nurse staffing and other components of hospital service. Therefore, one of the purposes of the book is to illuminate the nursing link between physicians and their hospital patients in order to enable physicians to participate more effectively in hospital quality-of-care efforts. High quality hospital nursing service improves the medical outcomes for patients, and it lowers the cost of hospital care. For this reason, this book focuses largely on nurses, the largest professional group in hospitals.

Like physicians, registered nurses are finding that the commercialization of their practice is increasingly placing them at the dictates of non-professional managers who view their practice, not as a professional process, but as a string of disjointed tasks. From these managers' accompanying perspective on nursing as a cost center rather than the revenue-producing service that it is, they are transforming nursing service into what logically seems to them to be a more economically efficient operation, that is, in effect, assembly-line "care."

As demanding as nursing school is, many graduates eventually abandon the profession to which they worked so hard to belong. Many of those who stay experience countless days dreading to report for duty. But the reason does not lie in the rigors of training and certainly not in the caring for patients. On the contrary, nurses generally find hope and happiness in caring for their patients. They are convinced of the value of their profession, and practicing that profession well enriches their lives, making the hard work and training worthwhile. Their profession has a rich history, which many believe is more altruistic than any other profession.

Nursing can be one of the most interesting and gratifying careers. What may appear to some to be a one-dimensional pursuit is inherently broadening and powerful, and it *requires* self-discovery. Nurses and doctors are consistently immersed in the most intimate struggles and celebrations of humankind, young and old, rich and poor and all other variations. On any given day, encounters with patients can be calm, even lighthearted, at one moment, then characterized by sheer terror the next. Under the most hurried and stressful circumstances, the accuracy and judgment of health professionals has to be at its peak. Nurses develop the art of prioritizing and organizing, often on a minute by minute basis, to a level that those outside their professional culture would find difficult to fathom. Practicing nurses quickly learn what they are made of, and those working with them do as well.

But it is not the challenges of nursing practice that destroy the spirits of nurses; it is working under conditions that *preclude* a professional practice. In some of our hospitals, it is impossible to provide good nursing care, no matter how good the practitioner may be.

The new hospital economy is also taking its toll on nursing education. Over sixty percent of nurses are now from associate-degree programs. Today's hospital economics encourages a more quickly-educated group at the bedside, lacking professional authority. Many of them enter nursing at an older age than that of nursing students in the past. Economics has become a more significant part of their training, and it should give us substantial reason for pause that many nurses who pursue their master's and doctorate degrees today do so, not in nursing, but in business.

One of the greatest barriers to improving hospital care has always been that others, including some physicians, have little understanding of nursing practice. Nurses' famous tradition of silence is partially responsible. True, nurses have been proclaiming the crucial relationship of their profession to the welfare of patients for some time. The problem is that they have not explained the *details* well. Explanations of nursing process are limited to nursing textbooks, while the public is barely aware that such a process exists, much less, how it critically affects their welfare as hospitalized patients. By in large, the public, as well as hospital managers and some health professionals, view bedside nursing care as a series of tasks and observations that admittedly require expertise but are mere tasks and observations nonetheless. Thus, patients, CEO's, physicians and even many of those nurses who have experienced little else consider it both acceptable and logical for hospitals to cut costs by hiring less expensive, non-professional assistants to perform so-called routine patient care tasks that supposedly require little skill and no judgment. This is the flaw in the perception of hospital nursing care that single-handedly prevents the success of serious attempts to improve hospital care quality, and it will do so even if budgets are increased.

While the so-called nursing shortage readily captures attention, nursing *practice* remains on the perimeter of serious hospital issues, which thwarts even the most labored and well-intentioned efforts to improve hospital quality and safety. All the while, the "nursing shortage" is, in reality, a shortage of *hospitals* where nurses can practice their profession as it is meant to be practiced. Currently, an estimated 500,000 RN's with active licenses (and an unknown number who have allowed their licenses to lapse) are not practicing. The most significant reason cited for this is the poor working conditions with which their community hospitals present them. There are another approximately 500,000 RN's who are working only part time.

If nurses and other professionals are to affirm their covenant with patients amid the obstacles in today's hospital climate, they will have to fortify their best qualities. Even when they disagree among themselves on any number of issues, they cannot disagree with regard to their essential professional values.

This book seeks to provide sustenance and encouragement to those professionals who would make it clear that the integrity of their practice is not for sale. It is written to benefit those who wish to understand and curtail a dangerously developing approach to hospital care before we have a new generation of nurses and physicians who simply don't know any better. It is not a your-nurse-is-the-one-who-really-takes-care-of-you book. Its purpose is not to enhance the status of nurses and certainly not to discount the essential roles of other professionals.

Nor is the book intended to berate already-beleaguered hospital CEO's. Achieving the difficult reconciliation of excellent care and profitability is a daunting responsibility. The need for economic survival places great pressure on CEO's to take what appears to be the safest management routes. An everyday work reality that distances them geographically and occupies them with details far removed from direct care and treatment of patients can easily disconnect even the most morally courageous CEO from the fundamental mission of care. With comfortable expertise in finance, yet little knowledge of their product, it is easy for CEO's to allow their focus to stray from the patient. Meanwhile, their highly educated and sometimes formidable "labor force" is just as likely to have the same knowledge and attention deficit regarding the financial realities of running the hospital.

Many individual hospital CEO's place a high value on patient care quality and on the needs of their community. They value the mission of the hospital. They understand the difference between management and leadership. They want to acquire an insight into healing and understand what they must do differently from other businesses when the product is care of the sick and injured. They understand that their most valuable resources are the human resources on their staff, and they want to facilitate excellence in these individuals. They would like to have their choice of the best of professionals, and they would like for those professionals to appreciate the importance of bottom line. They would like to overcome the chasm between themselves and those providing direct patient care at the bedside. This book supports those aspirations.

We all share the responsibility for creating hospitals we can trust. Despite objectives that are difficult to reconcile, professionals and executives must work together both to design good systems and to perpetuate the hospital's financial strength, producing a surplus for growth. Toward that end, the front office and the front line must value their complementary relationship. Meanwhile, the public must not allow themselves to be intimidated by what only appears to be a complex industry. They must be well informed enough to distinguish meaningful information from rhetoric and make reliable judgments about quality and the criteria for good care. They must examine the systems in their community hospitals, basing their efforts on the principle that good hospital care is best assured *before* one becomes a patient.

1

UNDERSTANDING
QUALITY HOSPITAL SERVICE

We rely on the substantial expertise of physicians to determine when we need to be in a hospital. Hospitals admit patients based on a physician's order. However, once we enter the hospital, much of the responsibility for our health, safety and dignity is placed in the hands of others. We may see our physician, even in ICU, no more than once or twice a day, during which time he or she determines the need for on-going diagnostic tests and medical treatments. It is nurses who are now the planners, coordinators and implementers of our care. In effect, the physician's judgment of whether we need to be hospitalized is inevitably based on our need for nursing service; otherwise, all treatments and surgical procedures could be accomplished on an out-patient basis. Even then, nurses usually guide the process.

It is a simple insight. Yet, the prevailing view is that nursing care is little more than a series of tasks, for which the technical simplicity or complexity alone determine the required level of the persons performing the tasks. That is, the more simple the task itself, the lower educational level required of the caregiver. As logical as this view appears, it is, in fact, the most important misconception about hospital care, and *it is the basis for public acceptance of poor service.* Nurses can even be made to believe it, given enough time and experience in hospitals where everyone around them perceives their role in that way and where working conditions leave them little choice but to practice accordingly. Increasingly, non-professional logic and self-interested rhetoric of others pervade and control the working environment of nurses, determining the character and quality of nursing practice.

It is crucial to the goals of this book that we first clarify the service we should expect when we enter a hospital. Therefore, the purpose of this chapter is simply to describe briefly the essential elements of professional nursing service for which we are paying, much of which may be surprisingly unfamiliar to the public. It then explains the conditions that must be present in order to render that professional service, making both economic and quality-of-care arguments.

THE ELEMENTS OF SERVICE

Most people are probably not even aware of the definition of professional nursing, which is the diagnosis and treatment of human responses to actual or potential health problems. This means that as nurses and doctors assist patients through the clinical process of healing, nursing is the profession additionally concerned with the individuality of patients and their circumstances. That is the independent function of nursing, accomplished by *nursing* diagnosis and treatment. For each patient, it requires an on-going assessment, a plan of care, the implementation of care and regular evaluation of care. Rather than a list of things to do, it is an individualized, professional process.

Nursing Diagnosis and Treatment

The public does not generally think of diagnosis and treatment as nursing functions. When nurses diagnose and treat patients, many people assume that they are crossing into the realm of medical practice, and sometimes they are. But a less familiar form of diagnosis and treatment, distinct from that of medicine, is essential to safe and competent hospital care.

Because it is different from medical diagnosis and treatment, there was much initial discussion within the nursing profession about whether to replace the terms with others that do not have physician/medical connotations. However, the terms stayed because they are accurate, distinguished from medical counterparts by their nursing focus.

There are also distinctions with regard to symptoms, etiologies and treatments. A medical diagnosis is based on symptoms that are usually constant from one patient to the next. For example, the physician is likely to diagnose diabetes if a patient presents the typical symptoms of headache, fatigue, excessive thirst, weight loss, blurred vision and elevated blood glucose level. Such symptoms are generally consistent in each patient with diabetes, regardless of personality, gender, age, cultural background, religious or political belief or any number of other individual differences. However, nursing diagnoses are often based on symptoms that vary according to the uniqueness of different patients.

If hospital nurses are to institute appropriate nursing measures for the diabetic patient, the nursing diagnosis must take into account everything that impacts the patient's management of the disease once the patient returns home. Can the patient self-administer insulin safely? Is their eyesight good enough to draw up an accurate dosage? If not, who will administer the patient's insulin? What cultural, intellectual, emotional or family influences affect compliance? An infinite variety of factors influence any patient's management of a chronic disease.

The premise of nursing diagnoses is the fact that patients with the same medical diagnosis may respond to the problem in decidedly individual ways. One patient who is admitted to ICU following a heart attack may be so frightened that they barely move or speak, while another patient in the same circumstances may be so frightened that he or she cannot be still or stop talking. In each case, the nursing diagnosis is the same, that is, anxiety. However, the nurse makes the determination from two opposite sets of symptoms because the two patients are different.

Naturally, other nursing diagnoses for these two patients will be the same, for example, activity intolerance, high risk for, or actual, cardiac arrhythmia or cardiogenic shock, and so on. But nurses frequently derive the same diagnoses from different symptoms, simple and complex, in different patients.

Just as symptoms may vary from one patient to the next, causes may vary as well, and nurses must tailor their treatment to the cause. For one heart attack patient, anxiety may result from a lack of information; for another, anxiety may result from too much information. The patient's fears may stem from anticipated decreases in future earning potential, the expected hospital and medical bills or any number of hidden worries. Pain causes anxiety as well, and vice versa. Just as there are various manifestations of anxiety, there are innumerable reasons for it, and in order to institute the appropriate nursing treatment, the patient's nurse has to discern the specific cause in each patient.

Appropriate nursing treatment requires individualized judgments and risk/benefit calculations, the consequences of which often appear deceptively minor in terms of successful patient outcomes. Relieving anxiety, for example, is not merely a nicety for patients, especially cardiac patients. Anxiety in such patients can easily have dire physiological consequences, such as precipitating major or even death-producing heart rhythms.

For patients with either acute or chronic illnesses, the medical diagnoses may remain the same throughout their hospital stay and require standard medical treatment. If the medical diagnosis is appendicitis, the treatment is appendectomy. If a patient has a respiratory infection, the medical treatment includes antibiotic therapy, administration of fluids, rest and relief of symptoms. If the patient has arthritis, the treatment may be medication, rehabilitation or surgery. Naturally, medical diagnoses are by no means always so straightforward. Even pathological processes in our bodies are individual. Still, in each case, the treatment, however complicated and demanding of the physician's judgment, is determined by the course of the disease itself.

But nursing diagnoses and treatments for the same patient may frequently change, either in accordance with or regardless of the medical condition. For every new mother with the medical diagnosis of "twenty-four hours postpartum," the nurse cannot assume the same set of nursing diagnoses. While all new mothers who are twenty-four hours postpartum may have some nursing diagnoses in common, such as risks of hemorrhage, they may or may not also have a knowledge deficit regarding how to care for themselves and their baby. Some may experience difficulty breast-feeding; others will not. Some may have ineffective coping, delayed bonding or other problems. Some may have infants who were born prematurely or have other complications, which will necessitate still other nursing measures. For all of these problems, the etiology and symptoms are highly individual; it follows that nursing measures will be highly individual.

Naturally, many patients with the same medical diagnosis will have *some* of the same nursing diagnoses. One of the nursing diagnoses immediately following the placement of a cardiac pacemaker is a risk for decreased cardiac output caused by a malfunction of the pacemaker or competition from the patient's natural rhythm. Although the degree of risk may be modified according to various factors, some interventions are basically the same for all patients: continuing assessment of heart rhythm, breathing pattern, blood pressure, skin color and lung sound. There are other nursing diagnoses and interventions common for all patients with newly implanted pacemakers.

The North American Nursing Diagnosis Association has approved over a hundred nursing diagnoses, and for readers who are interested in scanning the list, it appears at the end of this chapter. Individual nurses may elect to state other diagnoses as well.

Nursing treatment may or may not be the same for patients who have the same nursing diagnosis. Even seemingly insignificant individual preferences of patients and the nursing measures that honor those preferences may play a much larger role in patient outcomes than one might imagine. Any amount of control the patient can retain during a time when so much is out of their control is therapeutic. The degree to which some factors become significant is eminently influenced by illness, especially serious or chronic illness.

Thus, nursing is both a subjective and an objective process that requires a knowledge base very different from that of medicine. Given the endless range of conditions in which human patients find themselves and the significant impact of those conditions on healing, professional nursing at the bedside is the only appropriate means of delivering quality hospital service.

The Patient Assessment

Correct nursing diagnoses require both an initial and an on-going assessment throughout the patient's hospital stay. An initial assessment is generally a deliberate, systematic process involving the nurse's interview and physical examination of the patient as well as data from various other sources. Naturally, emergencies require a rapid analysis of symptoms, sometimes in a matter of seconds.

Assessment continues throughout the patient's hospitalization, often unnoticed, as the nurse cares for, directly observes, and communicates (both verbally and non-verbally) with patients and family members, physicians and support people. Whenever a nurse walks into a patient's room, whether to bathe the patient, to perform a complicated clinical procedure or to answer the patient's request for information about how to dial long distance on the bedside telephone, the nurse is processing observations and assessing the patient's condition.

A Plan of Care

Once the nurse completes the assessment and determines diagnoses, he or she writes an individualized care plan. Sometimes the nurse is justified in using a standard, pre-written care plan for patients with the same medical diagnosis, if this saves writing time. However, even the pre-written care plan allows for deleting unnecessary measures, and it presumes the addition of individual nursing diagnoses and treatments. It may change several times a day or several times a week as the patient's condition changes or as its effectiveness indicates.

The nurse bases the care plan not only on an analysis of patient symptoms but on an abundance of unique patient circumstances and needs, including medical treatments. It includes all current nursing diagnoses and treatments, complicated and otherwise. There are many simple comfort and peace-of-mind measures, easy to include in a well-designed plan, that promote the well being of patients and ease the minds of families.

The nurse writes the care plan using measurable goal statements such as, "Mr. Smith's lungs will be clear to auscultation within 24 hours" or "Ms. Brown's husband will correctly determine her blood glucose level and administer her insulin each morning for three days prior to her discharge from the hospital." If the nurse diagnoses a high risk for impaired skin integrity because of the patient's immobility or poor nutrition, the goal statement is, "Skin will remain intact, with no redness over bony areas." The approach to achieving the goal may read, "Change the patient's position, massaging the bony areas every two hours and offer an eight-ounce liquid protein supplement twice a day."

All nurses taking care of the patient use this care plan as their guide, regularly documenting its implementation and effectiveness. It allows for a systematic, well-coordinated, well-documented approach to each patient's care. It is the means of communication among all of the patient's nurses, thus providing continuity. It spares the patient and family the tiresome repetition of explanations and requests to nurses, and it spares nurses the unnecessary, time-and-energy-consuming activity of continuously reinventing the wheel. It also provides for the coordination of medical treatments and diagnostic tests, provides for as smooth and uncomplicated a hospital stay as possible for the patient, and it facilitates healing. It serves as a guide for discharge planning, and its use can shorten the patient's stay, which saves the hospital money.

Having realistic and well-designed care plans for each patient also benefits the nursing unit as a whole. Nursing unit coordinators can use care plans to make nurse/patient assignments according to unique skills, strengths and weakness of individual nurses, thereby utilizing the nursing staff most appropriately and efficiently. Rather than using the "warm body" (any licensed nurse will do) approach to staffing or making assignments according to geographical groups of patients (room 320 through 330), unit coordinators make their judgments based on the qualities of nurses that may make them best suited to the needs of particular patients. Furthermore, care plans are a guide to determine staffing overall and to justify requests for third-party reimbursements. Documentation is how hospitals are paid.

THE REQUIREMENTS FOR QUALITY

The professional care just described requires an organizational framework that allows it. That framework is characterized by: (1) a professional bedside nursing staff (2) a system of primary nursing (3) an appropriate nurse/patient ratio and (4) the elimination of non-nursing tasks from the responsibilities of nurses. All four of these elements are essential. When one is missing, it significantly compromises the other three.

A Professional Nursing Staff

An all-RN bedside nursing staff is not merely a luxury; it is a means of accelerating healing, reducing complications and lowering hospital costs. Having more registered nurses taking care of patients means fewer patient deaths, while utilizing nursing assistants, even for basic care, has correlated with increased patient complications. Aside from the obvious problems complications pose for the patient's health, they are very expensive developments.

The benefit to patients of an exclusively professional hospital staff extends beyond the fact that the most skilled and knowledgeable persons plan, coordinate and implement care. Many studies point to the additional value of collaborative nurse/physician relationships. Observation of clinical changes is far more likely to be sooner rather than later when the person directly caring for the patient has the ability to identify problems or potential problems before they become major.

Exclusively professional staffing also enhances patients' confidence in the hospital. Patients feel that they are in capable hands; they are likely to perceive their caretaker as competent and believe that their needs will be met. It follows that they will return to this hospital the next time they are seeking care.

Without a doubt, many nursing assistants are highly intelligent, kind and mature people who are quite reliable and have sought their jobs because they enjoy helping others. Almost any nurse will cite a particularly competent nursing assistant with whom the nurse would sometimes prefer working more than the nurse would prefer working with certain RN's.

But the character, integrity, emotional maturity and social skills of assistants vary widely, and their jobs are often much more difficult than they anticipated. The issue is not whether natural, personal qualities of some nursing assistants render them more competent (or more agreeable) than some nurses; the issue is about academic and clinical preparation. Basic skill training, with other important qualities left to chance, is not appropriate preparation for the complex care of acutely ill, hospitalized patients. It does not instill the observation and therapeutic communications skills that are essential in hospital caregivers. Furthermore, the training of nursing assistants does not prepare them for the pressures of their work or the tragic human drama to which they are often exposed in hospitals.

Unlike professionals, when nursing assistants make mistakes, they are less likely to realize it and less likely to understand the possible consequences for the patient. While the mistakes of professionals are usually related to inadequate staffing, unfamiliarity with patients or miscommunication, the mistakes of nursing assistants are characterized by the added factor of a lack of knowledge and poor judgment. Furthermore, non-professional workers may not always report their mistakes, especially when they do not appreciate the significance of the mistake to the patient.

One might assume that the simple work requirements of nursing assistants do not place them in a position to make serious mistakes, but nothing could be further from the truth. Some examples of mistakes made by nursing assistants are as follows:[1]

Drawing blood from the wrong patient, including a second time after the results of the first were questioned and the test repeated

Turning off a ventilator by mistake

Confusing an IV line with a tracheal line and drowning a patient

Inserting a urinary catheter that was two sizes too big for the patient

Causing the death of a patient by neglecting to return the head of the bed to an elevated position, allowing his lungs to fill with fluid

Mishandling an IV line and causing the death of a patient with an overdose of morphine

Sleeping at a cardiac monitor station while an alarm is beeping and a patient is dying

---

1. reprinted with permission from The Philadelphia Inquirer, June 6, 1997.)

We all make mistakes, sometimes under the best of circumstances. Still, even in poor working conditions, it would be extremely rare for a nurse to make any one of the mistakes listed. Since this report, the number of assistants has increased, not only in nursing, but in other departments as well.

Working with assistants can be a very stressful responsibility since one cannot usually supervise them directly. One nurse passed by a patient's room as two assistants were helping the patient dress. There is hardly a task that could be more simple. Yet, it caught the nurse's eye immediately that, in order to remove the patient's hospital gown, one of the assistants had temporarily disconnected the patient's IV line from the box that regulates its flow rate. With no visible change in demeanor, the nurse discreetly lunged in silent terror to clamp the open tubing that by then may well have allowed twenty-four to forty-eight hours' dosage of heparin[2] to be given in a matter of minutes!

The assistant was only doing what she had noticed nurses themselves do on occasion because in many cases, depending on the content of the IV fluid, it is perfectly okay to do so. In this instance, the nurse not only had to deal with a sudden critical development but she also had to do so while maintaining outward calm so that the patient would not realize the gravity of the situation and be frightened out of his wits. She also had to calm the nursing assistant who was horrified to learn the possible consequences of her action.

There is another important consideration with regard to nursing assistants and hospital mistakes. Nurses have traditionally been in a position to prevent many of the mistakes made by physicians, pharmacists, dietary workers and others, even laboratory technicians, because nurses are usually the last link to the patient. This has always been an understood function of nursing, and it diminishes considerably when nursing assistants are the last link to the patient.

---

2. Heparin is an intravenous medication that prevents the formation of blood clots. The calculation of its dosage and monitoring of its administration necessitate extreme care because an excessive dosage can cause hemorrhaging.

An all-RN staff is a means of both insuring quality and reducing staff. Contrary to what may seem logical to hospital managers without the professional training and experience of nurses, RN's can provide total care for patients more efficiently than a combination of RN's and nursing assistants can provide. The reduction in a need for coordination of activities, direction and instruction alone can save so much time that it more than makes up for the higher salaries of professionals. An all-RN staff further saves money by contributing to a reduction in personnel turnover wherever professionals experience the gratification that comes from an environment in which they are able to practice well.

It is true that nursing assistants tend to work competently and safely when a nurse is working with them. The problem is that most of the work done at the bedside does not require two people, so this is another waste of money. Nursing assistants also have a propensity to pair up with each other as they work and are thus more likely to chat among themselves rather than observe and communicate with the patient. They are more likely to find themselves in disputes with patients or families, for which the drain on the nurse's time and energy is also a cost factor.

The academic requirements for baccalaureate degree nurses are demanding, as is the process of specialty certification, and when those nurses practice at the bedside, their skills in assessment, diagnosis, implementation of care and evaluation are significant determinants of the most successful and least costly patient outcomes. The all-RN nursing unit is a significantly safer and clinically superior place for patients.

Primary Nursing

Marie Manthey[3], one of the first and most thorough authors on this subject, describes primary nursing as "the avenue to quality and humanization of

---

3. Manthey, Marie, The Practice of Primary Nursing, Blackwell Science, Inc., Boston, December 1980.

care in hospitals, the system which exemplifies nursing's purpose and transforms bureaucratic institutions into places where persons are respected and cared for as individuals." It is the system that most assures safe, competent and humane hospital care, both nursing *and* medical.

Primary nursing has been established for many years as the best system of hospital nursing care. It is a very simple concept, but it has important elements, none of which can be excluded. In her book, *The Practice of Primary Nursing*, Manthey describes its components, summarized below:

1. Throughout the patient's stay on a given unit, one nurse has the responsibility for that patient's care. Rather than a unit coordinator, charge nurse, case manager or any other person or "team" appointed to design care plans, the primary nurse is the decision-maker and the one who is held accountable. This nurse is also the implementer, that is, the hands-on doer of nursing care, and he or she decides what patient information is made available to whom. The patient and family, the physicians, other nurses and all with whom the primary nurse collaborates know that role. Typically, this nurse is on duty five days a week for eight-hour periods.

2. On the remaining shifts, other nurses caring for the patient follow the primary nurse's plan of care (unless changes in the patient's condition necessitate a different course). An associate nurse, who also remains constant throughout the patient's stay, is on duty on those days when the primary nurse is absent, which insures continuity and coordination of care. Associates may be primary nurses for other patients at the same time.

3. Charge nurses make *patient* assignments, not task assignments. The primary nurse then assumes all responsibility for those patients' care, from simple to complex. When the care requires a skill beyond the assigned nurse's level, it is that nurse's responsibility to see that someone who has the required preparation carries out the task.

Manthey describes the channels of communication as direct. Information is direct to and from the primary nurse, associate nurse, doctor, pharmacist, therapist, social worker and other necessary persons. It is not filtered through a pyramid or a team, resulting in a waste of time and the possibility of data distortion. Also, the nurse going off duty reports directly to the on-coming nurse during walking rounds, using the care plan. This allows the nurse visual assessment of the patient during the report, and it fosters good rapport with the patient and family. It also promotes confidentiality, and it is reassuring to patients that their care is well understood and communicated among their caregivers.

In the system Manthey describes, the responsibility of top and middle managers is more facilitative than directive. They determine appropriate nursing budgets, establish avenues for quality assessment and control, establish salary reward systems to promote the development of clinical competence and insure that nursing activity includes only that which falls into the realm of nursing practice. Non-nursing activities are the responsibility of support services. In general, the role of nursing managers is to maintain the organization and climate necessary to facilitate the best professional practice for bedside nurses.

Primary nursing allows for the best planning and organizing of patient-care activities, which can make a substantial difference in terms of cost and patient benefit. Nurses who are familiar with their patients can often administer medications and perform treatments in almost half the time that they can otherwise. Rather than several persons appearing at different times to perform various tasks, a primary nurse, well-acquainted with the patient's needs and routine, coordinates tasks more appropriately and efficiently, often during one visit to a patient's room. This decreases traffic, removes the need for incessant relaying of information and instructing among the staff and promotes a more tranquil atmosphere on the unit. It is understandably far less stressful for the patient, and because fewer persons have contact with the patient, it reduces the patient's risk of infection. This is particularly important for persons who have had surgery, for the elderly and for those with compromised immune systems. The coordination of care that characterizes primary nursing is *enormously efficient*, the least expensive system of nursing care in the long run, not to mention that it also eliminates the fees of non-nurse efficiency consultants often hired by major hospital corporations.

Although primary nursing, like any other system, requires an adequate nursing staff, it does not in itself require additional staff. On the contrary, it allows for maximum use of available professional nurses, and it saves money. As a former director of nursing, fully confronted with the realities of meeting the practical demands of nursing service, Manthey addresses scheduling details and costs. She instituted primary nursing in her own facility with no additional budget allowances.

Primary nursing also allows for the best complementary relationship between nursing practice and medical practice. It creates the natural process by which the nurse becomes a true partner who can collaborate effectively with physicians and others involved in the patient's care. Physicians and nurses may not necessarily operate from a colleague relationship (they are, after all, two different professions), but within the system of primary nursing, they will work together most effectively for the benefit of the patient. It is, in fact, the presence or absence of primary nursing that determines whether the nurse/physician relationship will be characterized by true professional collaboration or whether it will be nothing more than the physician-dictate variety.

Contrary to the sometimes negative image of the working relationship of doctors and nurses, almost all physicians relish quality input from nurses. In general, physicians do not discount the nurse's opinion when the nurse is familiar with the patient's case. That does not mean physicians always follow nurses' recommendations, though they often do, but they rarely dismiss them as inconsequential. Most physicians would like to have better working relationships with nurses if they could because when such relationships exist, both doctors and nurses feel better about their decisions and are more confident that they are doing the right things for their patient.

Primary nursing also promotes good relationships between nurses and families. Family members come to trust the hospital, as they see their loved one cared for directly by the same professional primary nurse and associate nurse throughout their stay. They become confident not only because the care is superior but also because they can see that these nurses are thoroughly familiar with the patient's needs and circumstances. Their nurses rarely mind being interrupted at lunch or being called at home. In fact, most primary nurses encourage family members or associate nurses to contact them about patient issues whenever they need to.

Another significant characteristic of primary nursing is that it makes the meaningful evaluation of an individual nurse's performance so easy. Accountability is built-in. Patient outcome and well being are high on the list of evaluation criteria, and the evaluator knows whose patient this is.

Enough Nurses

Many factors determine an appropriate nurse/patient ratio. It varies according to different nursing units within the hospital and changing patient acuity levels on the same unit. Sometimes it varies according to the time of day or night.

This is not a decision to be made by a non-nursing manager, based on numbers. Nurses themselves have tried to develop and use number systems for staffing, generally basing these systems on patient census and/or numerically designated patient acuity levels, and many nursing units are currently doing so. But the systems do not work well. The judgment of a nursing unit coordinator or charge nurse, taking into account all influencing factors, is the most reliable tool for determining RN/patient ratios at any given time (provided that "all influencing factors" do not include financial incentives to decrease staff).

In the presence of all of the other elements previously described as essential to competent hospital nursing practice, nursing managers can follow a *general guide* with regard to staffing. In units such as ICU or Obstetrics, the best ratio is one patient per nurse, night or day. Sometimes a nurse can safely care for two patients. On most non-ICU floors, the ratio is usually best at one nurse per four or five patients. These are only general rules, to which there are frequent exceptions.

It should also be noted that shifts should last only eight hours. Many hospitals institute twelve-hour shifts as a shortsighted means of cutting costs. While twelve hours may not be too long for some, it is too long for nurses, who must remain alert, accurate and physically active. An unsafe level of mental and physical fatigue begins to set in after eight hours, even among young nurses (the average age of practicing nurses is now forty-four) and under the best conditions.

Elimination of Non-nursing Responsibilities

On every nursing unit, there are many necessary secretarial and managerial tasks to attend, making it easy for managers to be caught in the pitfall of involving nurses in these tasks while nursing assistants take care of patients. At best, it is poor financial strategy to under-utilize professionals, even more so because the assistants who replace nurses make about the same salary as the secretaries the nurses are replacing! But the important consequence for patients is that it removes nurses from the bedside, focusing nurses' time and attention on extraneous details of the workings of the unit. Patients can only receive professional nursing care if professional nurses are taking care of them.

Eliminating these tasks for nurses is not an uncomplicated undertaking; it requires a deliberate and determined management approach and a specifically designed system. Naturally, it begins with distinguishing non-nursing tasks and separating them from the domain of nurses. It then requires the cooperation of other departments, such as pharmacies and laboratories, as well as secretaries and other support personnel. Nurses' stations must be designed so that individual desk spaces are away from telephones and the numerous other distractions. It is also necessary to establish a central communications unit to carry out the time-consuming task of processing physicians' orders.

*   *   *

These four hallmarks of quality hospital service – a primary nursing framework, an all-RN staff, an adequate number of RN's and the elimination of non-patient-care duties of professional nurses – are not an elusive ideal. They are the essential elements of hospital care for which patients are already paying, and they will most insure the best hospital course and outcome. They comprise a system that reduces patient complications and errors, shortens patient stays, decreases re-admissions and promotes patient privacy, dignity and confidence.

This is the service that also advances the financial goals of the hospital. Under the economic system of the moment by which government and the contract corporations for managed care reimburse hospitals, the hospital makes money if the patient leaves the hospital sooner and doesn't return shortly thereafter. Since healing is a process that depends heavily on quality of care, and good nursing care gets the sick person well in the shortest time, it stands to reason that quality nursing is crucial to the outcome for which hospitals are paid. The patient and family education that nurses provide has a direct relationship to the likelihood that patients will or will not do things wrong when they go home and thus, whether they will or will not end up having to come back to the hospital. The most financially responsible hospitals are those that provide the best nursing care they can.

Another economic reason for the best professional patient service is obvious from the drawers full of pending lawsuits one will find in hospitals at any given time. As patients and families become increasingly litigious, the cost that malpractice insurance adds to hospital care staggers the imagination.

Good service means not only that patients are far less likely to have cause for lawsuits but also that they are less inclined to sue, even when they have justification for doing so. Perceived competence of care and the respect with which patients are treated are strong determinants of whether they file lawsuits, even when things do not turn out as they should.

There is another economic benefit that generally escapes the notice of hospital managers. That is, an atmosphere that promotes quality also attracts nurses. Currently, only a minority of nurses are practicing at the bedside. What is referred to as a shortage of nurses might be stated as an abundance of nurses unwilling to practice in hospitals. A "solution" in recent years has been to offer sign-on bonuses to attract nurses. At this writing, one hospital offers a five thousand-dollar sign-on bonus, free day care *and* free lawn service. As attractive as the offer is, it is woefully misguided and shortsighted. The wrong solution to the wrong problem, logical only to those who understand neither. Ask any bedside nurse. Aside from a reasonable salary, a hospital need offer only *one thing* to its professional nursing staff: working conditions that allow good practice.

The expensive problem of turnover in hospitals and the scarcity of nurses are the result of (1) the many lateral career moves nurses make in search of an acceptable practice environment and (2) the large numbers of nurses who give up and leave the profession altogether.

Nurses want to be able to take good care of their patients. They want to practice their profession as it is meant to be practiced. A hospital that permits this will have an abundance of qualified applicants knocking at its door. It will not have to offer more money than other hospitals offer, nor will it have to offer sign-on bonuses or free lawn care of whatever else can be dreamed up in the minds of reality-detached managers and recruiters. The hospital that offers an environment in which nurses can provide safe, competent and professional care for patients will have its choice of the best of these professionals.

Nursing Diagnoses Approved by the North American Nursing Diagnosis Association:

activity intolerance
activity intolerance, high risk for
adjustment, impaired
airway clearance, ineffective
anxiety
aspiration, high risk for

body image disturbance
body temperature, altered, high risk for
bowel incontinence
breastfeeding, effective
breastfeeding, ineffective
breastfeeding, interrupted
breathing pattern, ineffective

cardiac output, decreased
caregiver role strain
caregiver role strain, high risk for
communication, impaired verbal
constipation
constipation, colonic
constipation, perceived
coping, defensive
coping, family: potential for growth
coping, ineffective family: compromised
coping, ineffective family: disabling
coping, ineffective individual

decisional conflict (specify)
denial, ineffective
diarrhea
disuse syndrome, high risk for
diversional activity deficit
dysreflexia

family process, altered
fatigue
fear
fluid volume deficit
fluid volume deficit, high risk for
fluid volume excess

grieving, anticipatory,
grieving, dysfunctional
growth and development, altered

health maintenance, altered
health-seeking behaviors, impaired
hopelessness
hyperthermia
hypothermia

incontinence, functional
incontinence, refex
incontinence, stress
incontinence, total
incontinence, urge
infant feeding pattern, ineffective
infection, high risk for
injury, high risk for

knowledge deficit (specify)

management of therapeutic regimen, ineffective
mobility, impaired physical

noncompliance (specify)
nutrition, altered: less than body requirements
nutrition, altered: more than body requirements
nutrition, altered: high risk for more (or less) than
body requirements

oral mucous membrane, altered

pain
pain, chronic
parental role conflict
parenting, altered
parenting, altered, high risk for
peripheral neurovascular dysfunction, high risk for
personal identity desturbance
poisoning, high risk for
post-trauma response
powerlessness
protection, altered

respiratory gas exchange
rape-trauma syndrome
rape-trauma syndrome: compound reactions
rape-trauma syndrome: silent reaction
relocation stress syndrome
role performance, altered

self-care deficit, bathing/hygiene
self-care deficit, dressing/grooming
self-care deficit, feeding
self-care deficit, toileting
self-esteem disturbance
self-esteem, chronic low
self-esteem, situational, low
self-mutilation, high risk for
sensory/perception alterations (specify visual, auditory, gustatory, tactile, kinesthetic, olfactory)
sexual dysfunction
sexuality patterns, altered
skin integrity, impaired
skin integrity, impaired, high risk for
sleep pattern disturbance
social interaction, impaired
social isolation
spiritual distress (distress of the human spirit)
suffocation, high risk for
swallowing, impaired

thermo-regulation, ineffective
thought process, altered
tissue integrity, impaired
tissue perfusion, altered (renal, cerebral, cardio-pulmonary, gastro-intestinal or peripheral)
trauma, high risk for

unilateral neglect
urinary elimination, altered patterns
urinary retention

ventilation, inability to sustain spontaneous ventilatory weaning process, dysfunctional violence, high risk: self-directed or directed at others

2

RECOGNIZING POOR SERVICE

Task-Oriented Care and the Impact on Quality

Hospital accrediting agencies do not insure quality patient care, nor do they claim to do so. They do not require the four conditions just described or that nursing work shifts be limited to eight hours. They require a minimal number of what is referred to as "licensed" persons, determined by the patient census, but they do not require consistency in patient assignments or that only "licensed" people provide patient care. They do not require the elimination of non-nursing functions from the responsibilities of bedside nurses. They do not require many of the conditions known to facilitate effective physician/nurse collaboration. They do audit patients' charts for some documentation of the nursing process, which is usually minimal and may insure only that the patient's chart, if not necessarily the patient, is the beneficiary of the nurse's expertise. Accrediting agencies also allow hospitals many months to prepare for their visits. In the end, they claim only to insure that hospitals are capable of providing a certain level of service, which is a tall order. But they do not insure professionally competent, safe and compassionate hospital care.

There are nursing frameworks in some hospitals that diminish the personhood of patients and compromise both their recovery and safety. These frameworks bear any number of labels that change from time to time, but they amount to task-oriented nursing, often referred to as functional nursing. It is a dark-ages system considered by the profession to be a relic of the past as modern nursing evolved. Unfortunately, it has vigorously resurfaced. Although the nursing profession abandoned it years ago as an inappropriate system of caring for the sick and injured in hospitals, some hospital managers are now touting it as the modern version of nursing that nurses, and therefore patients, will have to get used to. In reality, they do not understand their business well enough to operate a financially successful hospital that offers high quality.

Instead, they offer the mass production model of hospital care, involving an abundance of nursing assistants to perform so-called simple tasks and as few RN's as the accrediting agency will permit. Each RN has a long list of assigned patients and infrequent contact with patients. Meaningful collaboration between nurse and physician is minimal, and navigating the channels of communication is laborious and inefficient.

Within this framework, the head nurse, or unit coordinator, must regress to the difficult role of being the possessor of all knowledge. Since patients frequently change nurses, and nursing assistants provide much of the direct care, it falls to the head nurse to be the knowledgeable professional on the unit to which physicians, families and others must bring their questions and concerns.

Whenever hospitals place a mix of RN's and nursing assistants on their units, functional nursing is born. It is unavoidable. Patient assignments become task assignments, regardless of how they are characterized. First, patient assignments per nurse nearly double. One nurse and one nursing assistant (sometimes one-and-one-half or two assistants) may be responsible for eight, ten, or even more patients. One nurse cannot provide direct care for so many patients; the increased paperwork and documentation alone will prevent it, and if the hospital also requires that the nurse take on additional non-nursing, secretarial tasks, as is usually the case, the RN is even further removed from the patient's bedside. Consequently, the nurse focuses on the schedule of physician-prescribed medications, treatments and tests while depending on nursing assistants, out of sight, to provide patient care and observe for and recognize signs of change in patients' conditions. For nurses and assistants alike, care becomes little more than a series of unrelated tasks, no matter how much they would like it to be otherwise.

The nursing assistants may begin with a routine such as checking all the temperatures, blood pressures and pulses. Next, they go down the line giving baths. Then, they tackle the numerous other so-called routine tasks within the legal scope of their technical skills, such as checking all the blood glucose levels of the diabetics. Since such routines have little likelihood of coinciding with the individual timetables of patients' needs, patient call bells frequently interrupt the work.

Meanwhile, the nurse gives all the medications and does all the charting for the left side of the hall, as well as all other tasks ascribed to the "licensed" person. (In hospitals, the term "licensed person" is becoming a substitute for "nurse.") No matter how professionally competent the nurses are or how intense a responsibility they feel for their patients, this division of labor constitutes functional nursing.

Managers unencumbered with the professional knowledge, experience and responsibility of nurses may find it logical to assume that assembly-line nursing is efficient and therefore less expensive. That is not the case. Granted, most of the time, functional nursing gets the work done. Patients receive custodial care, and nurses carry out the physician-prescribed treatments, though probably with less accuracy. But any observer will be struck with the inefficiency of this system when compared to that previously described, especially when this system is also characterized by an inconsistency of nurse/patient assignments, causing nurses to care for patients with whom they are unfamiliar. The atmosphere on the unit is more hurried, and the activity is less coordinated. Even simple procedures can become complicated, requiring more trips back and forth down the hall to obtain supplies or assistance or to attend to interruptions, and the procedures can take longer to accomplish in the patient's room. Patient call bell use is more frequent because patients must make more requests even for routine care.

Functional nursing profoundly affects quality, with the primary emphasis necessarily on assisting the physician and getting the work done on schedule. Patient's family and visitors are all too often viewed as interferers with work (or as handy assistants). Unfortunately, fewer and fewer nurses have the benefit of ever having practiced in any other system, but those who have practiced primary nursing will readily affirm sharp contrasts between the quality of these two approaches to hospital care.

In many hospitals today, managers view the nurse merely as one who can legally perform a longer list of tasks than the assistants can perform. Furthermore, because nurses are handy and capable, they can also assume many non-patient-care duties, such as answering telephones, directing visitors, posting lab work, assisting hospital personnel and taking on a myriad of other secretarial or managerial tasks.

It is a system that eventually leads observers, including nursing assistants, to assume that nurses do not wish to be at the patient's bedside, that they think themselves above giving patient baths and providing other so-called low level patient care. For most nurses, that assumption is wrong. In fact, many ICU nurses say that one of the main reasons they prefer ICU nursing is that ICU is one of the few places in the hospital where they can give direct patient care. Separation from the patient (while still bearing responsibility for the patient) is what drives nurses to look for avenues open to them other than hospital nursing.

Both nurses and nursing assistants find their situations problematic. Assistants usually have a lot of work to do, but they feel little responsibility for the overall welfare of patients. The nurses must bear full responsibility for patients without the benefit of the patient contact than that responsibility requires. It takes little imagination to picture how routine and unrewarding the work becomes for nursing assistants and how stressful and unrewarding it becomes for nurses. It also sets up a relationship between nurses and assistants that easily creates resentment between them.

Next, imagine how this is manifested in their relationships with patients. At best, nursing assistants' heavy workloads tax their ability to convey friendliness. The assistant, who is likely to have fewer social (and coping) skills and has less than a professional, therapeutic approach to begin with, may well vent his or her anger and frustration on the most vulnerable person, the patient. The nurse, in an attempt to project professional concern for patients amid a sea of unrealistic responsibilities, all too often becomes one whose expression and countenance constantly change from caring professional to stressed assembly-line worker, depending upon whether he or she is in or out of the patients' view.

In such an atmosphere, there is a tendency to become more concerned with meeting legal requirements rather than meeting patients' true needs. All the while, the risk of lawsuits is extremely high because the system lends itself to errors and delayed recognition of important changes in the patient's condition. The care itself is of poor quality, and patients do not feel respected as individuals.

Nurses working in this system dread getting telephone calls at home; such calls are almost always for the purpose of informing them that something was not done right or asking them, usually at the last minute, to work extra shifts. Seldom is the purpose to discuss the best care for a particular patient.

In the absence of primary nursing, responsibility is obscure; when too many people are involved in the patient's care, and those people change from day to day, nobody is responsible for the patient. Family members may have the experience of wasting their breath explaining some bit of information to one nurse, only to be assigned the next day to another nurse who knows nothing about it. Lack of coordinated care and lack of familiarity because of inconsistent patient assignments is frustrating for both the patient and the nurse.

Patients, many of whom come into the hospital already lacking the important advantage of continuity in their medical care, face the same lack of continuity in their hospital nursing care. Increasing costs and interruptions in insurance coverage prevent many patients from having the long-standing relationship with their physician necessary not only for each to develop mutual rapport and trust but also for the physician to acquire the best medical history of the patient. When hospitalized, patients may then have different nurses each day. They transfer from one location to another within the hospital as their condition changes. The missing continuity jeopardizes both quality and safety.

If you are the patient, what you are likely to hear from the nurse is, "Mr. Smith, I'll be your nurse today," an introduction resembling that of your waiter. Thereafter, you seldom see "your nurse." Even the nursing assistants may change from day to day. It is not unusual for you to be cared for by an assistant from a temporary agency who may have barely worked in a hospital at all, if ever. "Your" nurse may not know your medical history and may need to refer to notes even for your current diagnosis. The nurse may never refer to your care plan, what there is of it, and having only the bare essentials to contribute, may discuss your case very little with the physician. Indeed, your nurse may well have to make an effort to recall which patient you are.

Very often, a patient's family member will stop by the nurses' station to talk with a nurse before leaving their loved one alone at the hospital. The family member explains one thing or another about the patient, pointing out that something in particular needs to be known or bears watching. No matter how responsive the nurse is, it is often easy to detect the family member's lack of confidence and the uneasiness they feel leaving their loved one alone in the hospital. Even if they believe that their family member is likely to be safe, which they sometimes do not, they rarely feel that the staff will meet the necessary needs in the best way.

Within this system, it is only natural that physicians may not even take note of which nurse is assigned to their patient. They have learned from experience that there is often little value in consulting with the nurse. Meanwhile, nurses often internalize that very self-image, even as they are scrambling heroically to get the work done and keep the floor running. No matter how heavy their responsibility, nurses' professional self-confidence and the confidence others have in them is consistently undermined amid conditions in which nurses have less information than others involved in the care of patients. (ICU's and a few specialized units are the exceptions, not because the nurses are different or better there, but because patient assignments are often more appropriate and consistent, and most of the time, RN's provide all of the direct patient care).

One of the most serious consequences of this problem, aside from undermining the confidence of an entire professional group, is the lack of physician/nurse collaboration. If the patient's nurse changes frequently, carries a large patient load along with a multitude of non-nursing responsibilities and gives very little direct care, then the nurse is not familiar enough with the patient to formulate the best nursing care plan or to contribute to that of the physician. Even when the physician looks to the nurse for substantive input, the nurse may have little or none to give. The nurse may not know whether the appearance of a wound is improved today over yesterday because a different nurse observed it yesterday. The nurse may have to refer to her notes even to recall the nature or location of the wound.

It is a natural consequence that doctor-dictate behavior sets in. The physician often communicates with the nurse simply by writing orders on the patient's chart or confining professional discussion to explaining how he or she would like something done. If another nurse will listen, the doctor would just as soon explain it to this nurse, trusting that it will be relayed to some appropriate person. In a system that consistently deprives them of effective professional collaboration, physicians understandably accept nursing care as little more than a series of tasks and a means of having their own orders carried out. It is not because they do not want a more professional relationship with the nurse but because they are accustomed to working without it.

Task-oriented nursing decreases quality considerably and has a profound impact on patient outcomes. Aside from depriving patients of the benefit of professional collaboration, the system places nurses in a position in which they are more likely to omit some of the observation and documentation of physician-requested data or overlook an aspect of the patient's routine care. Unfamiliarity with patients is one of the leading causes, if not the leading cause, of medication and other nursing errors.

The blame for all this is not only upon hospital managers who do not understand their product or with nurses who willingly submit to their authority. The problem is partly with physicians themselves because mangers sometimes consult them about nursing issues, such as staffing. CEO's, like so many others in the public and the media, assume physicians hold all knowledge related to health care, and when asked, many physicians give their opinions freely as though it were true. Physicians may tell CEO's what seems logical to them and, as it happens, it is also what CEO's want to hear, that is, that nurses are not needed to perform the more simple nursing tasks, and the hospital will save money by hiring non-professional persons for such work. Physicians then turn to nurses as though they've elevated the position of nurses and explain that this will free them to do the "real" nursing. It is an easy position to take when one does not understand what "real" nursing is.

Any nurse will attest to the fact that the seemingly simple task of bathing a patient provides the best opportunity to observe, teach and establish rapport with the patient. It is an important means of promoting healing, and it sometimes requires more clinical expertise and benefits the patient more than technically complex procedures. For that matter, there are strict procedures for bathing patients, in place for a reason, and assistants seldom follow them.

One physician-president, in support of changes he deemed appropriate in nursing service, remarked that it does not take a nursing degree to deliver a pill to a patient. With this statement, he illustrated not only ignorance of the professional nature of nursing but also thoughtlessness of what is involved in administering medicine. "To deliver a pill" has very broad patient-care ramifications, and it carries grave responsibility. Each nurse may administer over a hundred oral medications alone during a given shift, some of which are difficult for their acutely-ill patients to take and all of which require the nurse to understand indications, modes of actions, appropriate dosages, side effects and incompatibilities with other drugs or foods. An abundance of nursing textbooks focus on medications alone and the mathematical calculations often necessary to administer them correctly. It is one of the areas of their practice about which nurses feel the strongest responsibility for knowledge, accuracy and insight into their patients' diagnoses and problems. Imagine this physician's objection if confronted with the same flippancy on the subject of prescribing the pill.

Physicians are experts only with regard to their own profession. They are not nurses. Their education and training is different from that of nurses; medical practice and nursing practice are two entirely different professions. For one profession to define the practice of another is both illogical and arrogant. Hospital managers should consult nurses on nursing matters, and they should hire nurse assistants *only* for non-patient-care purposes, such as secretarial work.

The American Medical Association has not been a strong supporter of reforms proposed by nurses. Some observers say it is because physicians are looking out for their own self-interests, and they fear the potential power of nurses. Perhaps that is at least part of the reason. But it is just as likely that physicians simply have too little understanding of the professional nursing process and a lack of confidence in nurses, based on less-than-optimum collaboration with them.

Another casualty of functional nursing is the substantive, carefully designed and individualized patient care plan. Accrediting agencies require a care plan for each patient, but in functional nursing, it is likely to be of the bare bones variety, and nurses seldom refer to it, except to insure the required documentation, which itself is often neglected until the patient's discharge.

In functional nursing, nurses have four sources of information about their patients:

(1) The verbal or taped report given at the nurses' desk by the nurse going off duty. The on-coming nurses and assistants take notes from this report, and it is often given in earshot of, or directly to, other hospital personnel. There could easily be persons not involved with the patient's care listening to the report. Admittedly, the report rarely omits information necessary to the patient's immediate medical treatment and safety. However, such attention by itself does not constitute professional nursing care.

(2) The kardex, which is a computer file or a large index-type file of individual patient cards that list the room, diagnosis, age, current treatment (other than medication), current diagnostic testing, diet, activity level, and other basic information. It remains at the nurses' desk, and nurses use it as they are giving or receiving report. They refer to it any number of times during their shift and erase information as it ceases to be current. It is not a nursing care plan.

(3) The medication profile that nurses use for reference and documentation when administering medication. There are a number of protocols within the hospital to which nurses strictly adhere, and the procedure for administering and recording medications is necessarily one of them. This applies even to the simplest medications that could be purchased over-the-counter.

(4) The patient's medical record (chart) that nurses, physicians and various other professionals use for communication, reference and documentation.

The means of dispensing information to the nurse differs with functional nursing and primary nursing. Primary nursing also utilizes these four sources of information, in addition to others, but it differs with regard to the manner in which the report is given. In primary nursing, the nurse going off duty reports during walking rounds to the on-coming nurse and refers to the care plan. In functional nursing, the nurse focuses on minimal information and physician-prescribed treatments, medications, and diagnostic studies. They are likely to discuss other patient issues only on an informal basis, not as part of a systematic, deliberate approach to the patient's holistic care. Nursing diagnosis and treatment and a care plan take a distant back seat.

It is fascinating to observe the ever-more-inventive ways nurse managers devise for staff nurses to document so that professional nursing process will appear alive and well, when in practice it is hanging by a thread. The nursing care plan often amounts to a photocopied standard care plan for all patients with a given medical diagnosis, and it is merely additional paperwork. Upon the patient's admission to the hospital, the nurse glances through it quickly, placing a few checks, dates and initials, then places it on the chart, abandoning it until the patient is discharged, at which time the nurse insures that any final checks, dates and initials are in place.

Even excellent nurses cannot compensate for a poor system. They may have abundant energy, knowledge and competence, and they may possess the ability to comfort and instill confidence in patients. They may hold their own with physicians, even when they are barely familiar with the patient. They may inspire and work well with nursing assistants. They may be the best among their peers. As primary nurses, their value to the patient and family throughout hospitalization is incalculable. As functional nurses, their value to the patient lasts only for the duration of their shift.

REALITY VS. RHETORIC

Few self-respecting hospitals will own up to the practice of this assembly-line nursing, even as their RN/nursing assistant/patient ratios and their patient assignment patterns preclude any other way for their nurses to practice. If you ask hospital officials (including nursing unit coordinators who are expected to support the hospital's position) whether they have primary nursing, you are likely to receive one of a variety of responses:

> "We tried primary nursing, but it did not work for us."
> "Primary nursing isn't necessary for good care; good nurses are."
> "We try to maintain consistency of patient assignments."
> "Some of our units do not lend themselves to primary nursing."
> "We have a variation of primary nursing."
> "Primary nursing is not feasible in today's hospital economy."
> "We don't use primary nursing specifically; we use the (some other) system, and we provide high quality care."

All such responses mean "no." When hospitals say that they utilize a "variation of primary nursing," what they often mean is that they generally attempt to have some consistency in assignments. They still utilize nursing assistants, and their RN's may still have a multitude of responsibilities other than taking care of patients. An attempt at consistency of assignments is better than otherwise, but it is not primary nursing.

Other hospital managers claim to have primary nursing when in fact they do not. Again, they may have some consistency in assignments, but that does not suffice. Those who say, "We tried primary nursing, but it did not work for us," in fact, probably "tried" only some element of the system, or they fell short in the strict commitment that primary nursing requires.

As simple as primary nursing is, those implementing it must be consistently alert and committed. They must understand its premises and incorporate *all* of its integral parts every day. Otherwise, it will indeed "not work for us." How can one nurse be held accountable, for example, if he or she is only the "primary nurse" part of the time? At the very least, there goes the method of evaluating this nurse based on patient outcome. How can the unit coordinator refer the physician's questions to the patient's nurse, expecting full professional collaboration? Hospitals cannot claim they have primary nursing if nursing assistants are taking care of patients and nurses are assisting the secretaries.

One cannot determine whether hospitals have primary nursing or any of the other components of a professional system simply by asking. Public relations rhetoric often seems plausible, and it can obscure the facts. For that reason, it is important that inquirers be able to discern for themselves the four requirements of a quality hospital care system: primary nursing, an all-RN staff, an appropriate nurse/patient ratio, and the exclusion of non-nursing tasks from the responsibilities of nurses. A hospital either meets these requirements or it doesn't. Omitting even one of these requirements substantially compromises the benefits of the other three.

For someone who wishes to evaluate the hospital care in their community or on a specific unit in their hospital (systems may vary on different nursing units within the same facility), it is simple to determine the presence or absence of these necessary components of professional nursing service. Ask these three questions:

1. What are the credentials of each person currently working, part time and full time, on the unit? The presence of nursing assistants equates to a task-oriented system and distance between nurses and patients. This is true if each nurse is working with even one nursing assistant.

2. How many patients are assigned to each RN? One cannot realistically establish an inflexible nurse/patient ratio; however, the best *general* rule is to assign each RN to one, sometimes two, patients in ICU and Obstetrics and four or five patients on most other units.

3. May I see the patient assignments for the previous two weeks? This will reveal whether patients maintain the same nurse and nurse associate throughout their stay on the unit. It will also reveal whether nurses are on duty for more than eight hours. Without betraying confidentiality, the hospital can identify patients by assigned numbers, and if they like, they can also omit the names of their nurses

and assistants, listing them only according to credentials and assigned numbers.

Essentially, those are the only questions one need ask. But inquirers may also seek other information, such as the hospital's continuing education record for each nurse. Accrediting agencies may only require a yearly class on CPR, fire safety and infection control. Many state boards also require a minimum number of continuing education hours, but these are only minimum requirements, and some nurses acquire more. Ask how many of the nurses on a given unit are certified in that specialty and the amount of nurses' salary increase upon certification. Ask how much of each nurse's non-required continuing education and travel expenses were paid by the hospital during the past year. Many hospitals have significantly reduced their allowance for nurses' continuing education. It would also be enlightening to know how many of the nurses subscribe to a professional journal or belong to a professional organization. Functional nurses, especially those not practicing on a specialty unit, are not as likely to be motivated to do either.

These are simple, on-target criteria for anticipating the quality of service in any acute-care hospital. The inquiry does not ask hospitals to disclose confidential patient or employee information. If the news media would truly serve the public with regard to health care, they would focus their reports on these essential aspects of the hospital service in our communities, just as they focus on technology and the development of new drugs.

For individual patients and family members already hospitalized, it is too late to confront these issues. However, one may ask the caregiver whether they are a registered nurse, whether they are the primary nurse for the duration, how many patients they are responsible for and whether nursing assistants will be providing much of the bedside care. At least, the patient and family will then know whether the high price they are paying for hospital care is used for that purpose or whether their money is being spent elsewhere.

With the exception of some ICU's and specialty units, many such inquiries into the quality of service at our hospitals will be disappointing. Those hospital officials will claim that the expense is prohibitive, to which the inquirer has only to respond by asking the basis for such a claim because in reality, their claim is only an assumption. Given the fact that the described components have been designated by the experts, that is, nurses, as the working conditions required for their practice and given the significant theoretical economic benefits, has the hospital required, encouraged, or allowed even one nursing unit the opportunity to demonstrate the benefits? Have nurse managers requested the opportunity?

By instituting a carefully planned and appropriately implemented system over a specified period on one unit, the hospital could determine a wide range of business implications. Yet, hospitals do not experiment because nurses do not request it, because CEO's and managers do not understand the nature of their service or because the results might not show promise by next Thursday's corporate staff meeting.

A PERILOUS PATH

What we thought was nursing of the past is fast becoming nursing of the future in many hospitals. Some hospital officials have been saying that it's time to "re-evaluate the role of nurses" At a time when patients must be sicker than ever to qualify for hospital admission, what these persons are proposing and what has now been implemented in many hospitals across the country, however they may characterize it, is a return to functional nursing. Such systems of nursing are not "modern versions of the nurse's job," they are primitive, costly and often dangerous substitutes. They diminish the professional confidence of nurses, rob physicians of effective collaboration and rob patients and families of the medical and nursing care they need and for which they are paying.

Anyone admitted to a hospital submits to whatever level of quality that hospital provides. If nursing service is lacking, it compromises care for *all* patients. Poor and wealthy alike may well receive the same lower quality hospital care that has been described.

Hospitals are expensive enterprises, to be sure. Some are struggling to survive. Still, many hospitals squander resources on ineffective systems, inept or useless management, excessive salaries and bonuses for executives, excessive travel and entertainment, and unimaginable malpractice insurance costs to cover thousands of avoidable lawsuits. Such extravagant spending is listed as "operating costs," not profits. The millions of dollars paid yearly to a few corporate executives alone would hire an abundance of nurses. The same may be true for so-called non-profit hospitals as well.

Today many nurses have come to believe that primary nursing, all-RN staffs and the other components of a good system are impossible dreams: they are the ideal; therefore, we cannot have them. In the present economic environment, many nurses no longer dare to bring up the subject. They have gradually acquired very limited professional vision. Instead, they stand by while misinformed or self-interested outsiders determine their destiny, which is inappropriate for any profession. Meanwhile, bedside care is increasingly characterized by a string of bare-essential tasks doled out according to technical skill level.

Hospital officials will often try to convey the impression that to do otherwise is an expensive nicety. According to one, "Often the level of TLC that a patient expects – the back rub, the hand holding – doesn't get done in today's intense environment. But I don't think there is any evidence that the quality of hospital care has deteriorated." This deplorable reference to professional nursing as insignificant TLC is typical of the rhetoric coming from many hospitals officials today.

For a more realistic perspective, one has only to observe the patient who has lost hope and dignity or is locked in the grip of overwhelming anxiety or anger. Or consider the persons whose hospitalization or infirmity has been extended because of errors, complications, missed observations or neglected nursing diagnoses and interventions. Ask the courtroom plaintiffs who have lost loved ones.

The hospital official's remark exemplifies the lack of insight of many hospital managers into the complex process of healing and the crucial role of the nurse at the bedside. They dismiss the avenue by which nurses and physicians most effectively collaborate, and they expose their ignorance of the significance of that collaboration to their hospital's mortality rates, incidences of complications, lengths of patient stays, and other success or failure indicators, including the hospital's reputation, marketability and profitability. Either that, or they profess such opinions to deceive the public and advance self-interests. On some level, they may fear that their own role is far less essential than that of the person taking care of the patient.

There are determined and innovative CEO's who have led their hospitals successfully, maintaining both high quality service and the financial capacity for on-going modernization and expansion. Yet, in some hospitals, the leadership lacks the knowledge, integrity or will to enable their facilities to remain viable except by cutting immediate costs at the bedside, replacing patient care with the faceless performance of assembly-line tasks. It is an inhumane, dangerous and deceptively expensive approach, no matter how much the short-term cost reduction or how accompanied it is by a deluge of public relations rhetoric. Many of the hospitals that are failing are not doing so because they are impossible business enterprises; they are failing because they don't take care of their patients.

3

THE NEW URGENCY OF OLD ISSUES

THE NURSE/PHYSICIAN TEAM

As any discipline evolves, its members generally engage in on-going debate about the best way to proceed. Nursing and medicine are among the most recognized examples. One subject of debate has always been the complementary roles of nurses and physicians and how those roles change over time.

As the two professions have dealt with this issue, the result has been that nurses increasingly assume responsibilities that traditionally belonged to physicians. This is particularly true in intensive care and specialty units, and it has evolved, not because nurses were put-upon, but because achieving successful patient outcomes required it. Many lives have been saved, especially in ICU, where the stakes are raised.

Today, however, a new variable has entered the equation, creating risks in the established approach that was devised by professionals and heretofore working well. Cost cutting at the level of service and poor systems for nursing in many hospitals make it harder for nurses not only to provide safely for traditional nursing service but also to take on today's added responsibility for medical decisions.

To comprehend the gravity of this professional issue, it is necessary to understand the basis for ICU's and to note some of the specific responsibilities that nurses have gradually acquired. It is also necessary to understand how nurses and physicians had worked together to make their changing relationship advantageous to the patient and acceptable to the law.

From the beginning, intensive care units were extraordinarily successful, but they were not based on new technology. The technology utilized in these units had long been available. ICU's were a new system of *nursing*, one that almost immediately reduced the mortality rate of hospitalized victims of heart attacks, for example, by *thirty to forty per-cent!*

Because ICU's were revolutionary and successful in caring for critically ill patients, hospitals have traditionally supplied them with ample resources in equipment, professional staff and opportunities for continuing education. With such working conditions, nursing care and nurse/physician collaboration was of very good quality. Physicians came to expect a high level of competence among the nurses as a matter of course. In fact, some physicians struggled to measure up.

In order for ICU's to work, nurses had to take certain actions quickly without consulting the physician first. A common example involves heart rhythm irregularities, or cardiac arrhythmias, that frequently occur in patients during the first few days following a heart attack and must be diagnosed and treated immediately. The nurse apprises the physician after the fact, either right away or later during rounds, depending on the nurse's judgment of the need.

Today, medical diagnosis and treatment by nurses has expanded even further and includes numerous scenarios, both emergency and non-emergency. Patients in all ICU's, from pediatrics to burn units, may have conditions which change second by second, and it is not in the patient's best interest, indeed it is not at all feasible, for nurses to discuss each development with the physician before treating problems. This nursing approach continues to be the basis for the success of ICU's. Nurses sometimes engage in such diagnosis and treatment on general medical and surgical units also, though far less routinely.

To meet the requirements of the law, either nurses or physicians write a list of "Physician's Standing Orders," which they regularly review and update. The list is generally a full page or longer and includes whatever diagnosis and treatment initiatives the ICU nurses need in order to provide for a patient's best treatment during his or her stay in the unit. There are often several lists of standing orders for various purposes in one ICU, and nurses place the list/s applicable for a given patient on the chart when the patient arrives on the unit.

The physician fills in a blank or places a check next to those standing orders he or she authorizes. The physician may hand-write other orders according to patients' individual needs, but standing orders often make up the bulk of orders for an ICU patient, and occasionally, they are the only orders. Physicians may order other treatments or medications in any number of doses, to be administered at specified times or at the discretion of the nurse. Nurses embrace this practice because it clearly benefits the patient. Some physicians say they have very little doctoring to do in ICU because the nurses take care of the patients.

By authorizing standing orders, physicians are not necessarily directing the patient's care, nor are they supervising nurses. In such situations, both physicians and nurses are each directly responsible for medical diagnosis and treatment. A common example is the judgment ICU nurses must make about when to remove patients from artificial ventilation, that is, a ventilator or respirator used for patients when they are unable to breathe adequately on their own. Among the standing orders for post-operative open heart surgery may be one which reads:

Begin weaning (from the ventilator) when:

1. Patient awake and responsive

2. Stable hemodynamics

3. Good respiratory effort

4. Acceptable arterial blood gases on 40% oxygen or less

5. Bleeding <100cc/hr.

Given the above order, it is, in effect, the nurse's decision when to take a patient off the ventilator. All of the criteria listed are simply those that physicians themselves use, and analyzing the criteria involves medical expertise. An assessment of "stable hemodynamics" requires analysis of a combination of laboratory values, vital signs and other clinical symptoms. "Patient awake and responsive" requires judgment concerning the level of responsiveness and how well it is sustained. Judging acceptable arterial blood gases involves determining when to order the necessary lab work, analyzing a group of values and deciding whether together they are acceptable for the individual patient. Both nurses and physicians are also likely to rely on the judgment of the patient's respiratory therapist.

Heart rhythm disturbances are other events that require nurses to make medical diagnoses and institute medical treatments. Among the many kinds of rhythm disturbances that may occur are PVC's, premature ventricular contractions. It is often crucial to detect and correctly diagnose these irregular beats from the bedside electrocardiogram and treat them appropriately. Thus, the order reads:

1. If 6 or more PVC's/min., multifocal PVC's, PVC's on T, short bursts of 2 or more PVC's, administer lidocaine 1 mg./kg. IV push.
2. If ectopy persists, give 0.5 mg./kg. IV push 5 minutes later. Start lidocaine IV drip.

PVC's are common and often harmless, but when they occur in a patient who has just suffered a heart attack, they are taken very seriously. It is not at all uncommon for PVC's to be immediate forerunners of major or death-producing arrhythmias requiring electric countershock (defibrillation). If the nurse delayed in recognizing and treating this arrhythmia, if she took time to locate and consult the patient's physician, then more serious arrhythmias could develop quickly, and the patient could even die.

No physician is supervising this situation. It is the nurse who is making a medical diagnosis and deciding on a medical treatment. The standing order may appear to spell out exactly what decisions the nurse is to make, but it does not. PVC's are not always easy to diagnose. They are among about thirty or so other basic arrhythmias that may develop in the days following a heart attack, each requiring different treatment. Well-prepared, experienced practitioners, physicians or nurses, can be easily mistaken about arrhythmias. One may be quite difficult to discern from another, each requiring crucial differences in medication or treatment. Combinations of arrhythmias may occur. They may also occur for any number of reasons, requiring any number of approaches to their treatment, and so on. Knowledge of arrhythmias requires extended training. It also requires about a year's good experience to be able to diagnose most of them accurately and make judgments about their treatment. Treatment may then include medication, electro-cardioversion, the use of a cardiac pacemaker or other measures, none of which are likely to have minor consequences, and all of which may be instituted solely at the nurse's discretion.

Today, one of the treatments for heart attacks is to administer streptokinase or a similar "clot-buster" drug to help dissolve the clot obstructing the coronary artery. (A few years ago, only drugs that could inhibit further clot formation were in use: they could not dissolve or prevent damage from the clot that had already formed). The news media publicized these drugs, and rightly so, because they were a milestone in the treatment of heart attacks. However, to be effective, they must be administered within a certain time after the heart attack occurs. Furthermore, to be candidates for treatment with them, patients must meet specific criteria and undergo extremely careful monitoring as the drug is given. Drugs that dissolve clots can also cause hemorrhaging.

From the news accounts, it appears that physicians alone decide whether to use one of these drugs, they themselves administer it, and they stand by closely monitoring the patient first hand. They do not. It is usually the patient's nurse who makes this decision, administers the drug and monitors the patient. When a heart attack patient arrives in ICU, the nurse assesses whether he or she is a candidate to receive the drug. The nurse then informs the physician who, often acting solely on the nurse's judgment, responds with an "okay" to administer or withhold the drug.

These are only a few of the innumerable examples of medical judgments required by nurses. Standing orders simply list what physicians would do and the criteria they themselves would use to make decisions if they were present. Almost all physicians use them for their ICU patients. With standing orders, the physician is saying to the nurse, in effect, "You make the diagnosis and institute the appropriate treatment."

In addition to independent medical diagnosis and treatment, nurses often make suggestions to doctors. Years ago, both diplomacy and subtlety usually accompanied such suggestions so that they would seem to be the physician's idea. Diplomacy never goes out of style, but game-playing is seldom necessary today because many of today's physicians trained in ICU's with experienced, well-prepared nurses, and as young interns, the physicians became accustomed to looking to these nurses for advice. Physicians acknowledge that nurses spend much more time with the patient, and they frequently acquiesce to the ICU nurse's opinion.

The cooperative and collaborative relationship of hospital nurses and physicians is evident when one needs the other. Nurses will stop whatever they're doing if possible to consult with or assist a requesting physician. Similarly, whenever a hospital nurse (ICU or otherwise) needs to consult with the physician, he or she is almost always immediately available to the nurse. If the physician is away from the hospital or with an office patient, a nurse who telephones does not have to wait for a return call; the physician comes to the phone. Except during off-duty hours when a partner is taking calls, the physician either carries a beeper or informs the necessary hospital nurses of his or her location and telephone number.

Before telephoning a physician regarding a patient, the nurse usually anticipates the orders, if any. Many nurses jot those expected orders on a note pad in front of them before they dial, so they will be sure they have either gotten everything they were looking for or received a satisfactory explanation. This means only that these nurses are well prepared for thoughtful and productive communication. They generally do not second-guess a physician's course of action unless they believe it is clearly wrong for the patient, which it usually isn't.

Specialty units are similar to ICU's in many ways. Obstetric nurses, for example, commonly make medical diagnoses and institute medical treatments. It may be surprising to some to learn the extent to which this takes place, regardless of whether the patient delivers normally or has complications. For most obstetric patients, nurses employ standing orders just as ICU nurses do. These orders pertain to fetal monitoring, requesting lab studies, performing sterile vaginal exams, administering IV fluid, oxygen or pain medication and taking other measures deemed necessary for individual patients.

Often, it is the nurse who decides whether to administer intravenous pitocin, a drug that initiates or accelerates labor by causing the uterine muscles to contract. The nurse also decides the dosage, rate and duration of administration, all according to the progress and pattern of labor, the condition of the cervix, the baby's heart rate or some other factor.

Again, making such decisions is not simple. The use of pitocin has its dangers, such as the possibility of rupturing the uterus. It could also overstimulate the uterus, causing a deceleration in fetal heart rate. If the uterine muscles contract too intensely, blood flow cannot pass through to the placenta and fetal death can occur. An obstetric nurse has two patients, mother and baby.

Nurses consult with doctors via telephone regarding the patient's readiness for an epidural, the patient's blood pressure, the need for further pain medication, the need for a C-section, and other developments. As in ICU, the nurse has usually decided beforehand what course of action needs to be taken.

Expectant parents often seek nurse midwives, maintaining access to an obstetrician "in case something happens." The fact is, however, hospital obstetric nurses regularly handle complications. The obstetrician and the nurse together usually attend the mother when she delivers her baby. But the patient's labor, complicated or not, is often completely managed according to the judgment of the patient's nurse, even when there is consultation with the physician by phone. It is not unusual for nurses alone to attend the mother when she delivers, though most nurses predict the time of delivery closely enough to have the obstetrician present at that time.

One nurse recalled a patient who arrived unexpectedly on the unit. The nurses determined that a breech delivery was imminent, posing a potential danger to the baby. The patient's obstetrician could not be located quickly enough, and an ER physician was summoned. As he arrived, he immediately requested an experienced labor and delivery nurse. When she came, he said to her, "You deliver this baby and I will assist you." The nurse did so, and what is referred to on OB as a "good baby" was delivered.

ER physicians often must treat patients who have problems requiring a specialist not immediately available, except by telephone. They must use the best judgment they can under the circumstances, and in this instance, the best judgment was to depend on an experienced OB nurse.

In the hospital, procedures generally performed only by the physician are as follows:

1. The delivery itself, though the nurses at times find themselves in the position when they alone assist the patient with delivery

2. An amniocentesis

3. The rupture of membranes (breaking the water)

4. The epidural anesthesia, which is done by an anesthesiologist or a specially trained nurse anesthetist.

Nurses prepare the patients and attend them during and after those procedures. For example, in accordance with standing orders after a patient has an epidural anesthetic, the nurse stays with her to check blood pressure every five minutes for twenty minutes and observe for other signs that the procedure has gone well and the mother and baby suffer no ill effect. In the rare event that the epidural catheter was not placed correctly, the anesthesia could get into the blood stream, at which point it becomes systemic, not local, and places the patient at risk for a drop in blood pressure, difficulty breathing, or even respiratory or cardiac arrest. If it becomes a spinal anesthetic, the baby is at risk. Nurses consult with the physician whenever it is necessary for any reason, but just as with ICU nurses, there are times when resolving the matter at hand comes first and telephoning the physician comes second.

These descriptions are meant neither to minimize the role of physicians nor to exaggerate the role of nurses; they are merely a realistic portrayal of hospital care, particularly in ICU's and specialty units. In truth, the reality of the working relationship of doctors and nurses is easily revealed when a dire situation suddenly develops. If the patient's doctor is at the bedside, what you hear coming from the room is, "I need a nurse in here *now!*" Then again, if it is the nurse at the bedside, you may hear, "I need the doctor in here *now!*" The two professions are a team. Although the word "team," when used in other contexts, is sometimes tossed about loosely, it truly applies to nurses and physicians working well together in these settings.

THE TEAM AT RISK

Professionals have acknowledged and discussed these issues for years. Whether or not nurses are capable of fulfilling the roles of both collaborators and independent practitioners who make both nursing and medical judgments is not at question; they have been doing so for a long time, and their role in this capacity has served the patient exceedingly well.

Even so, one of the long-standing questions is whether they need more preparation. Physicians receive a generous (and expensive) education, yet the levels of education and experience of nurses vary widely. A baccalaureate program, and certainly an associate-degree program, by themselves do not adequately prepare nurses for the responsibilities they assume in ICU's. Nurses usually develop competence and expertise over time through their own private study, continuing education and experience on the unit. Today they may become certified in any number of specialties, but they are required to have about two years' experience in that specialty to qualify for certification examinations. In the meantime, they assume full responsibilities on their unit.

Another issue is whether ICU's should have a physician on staff twenty-four hours a day, as most Emergency Rooms now have. This may be one of the trends, though smaller community hospitals may be a long time in acquiring these physicians. Also, the addition of physicians to full-time hospital staffs significantly increases ICU costs.

There is another reason nurses have continually assessed their role in ICU's. They want to draw appropriate lines between assuming medical responsibilities that are truly necessary and those that are merely a means of making life easier for doctors. Nurses ask themselves, "Are we assuming these responsibilities because we can't find our way out of the physician's assistant role? Do we perceive the medical role as more interesting and more gratifying or having more status than the nursing role has? If so, are we willing to accept such supposed status in lieu of more appropriate salaries for the services we are performing?"

The fact that the public is largely unaware of nurses' roles in these units is another issue. It is difficult to carry such heavy responsibility in anonymity, downplaying the significance of one's own profession and perpetuating the importance and financial success of another. Many nursing issues eventually find themselves related to nurses' long-held tradition of silence.

Above all other issues, probably the most crucial for nurses has been the quality of their own practice. They ask themselves, "As we engage in medical practice, are we neglecting *nursing* practice? While we are diagnosing third degree atrio-ventricular block or atrial tachycardia and prescribing and administering intravenous medications, while we are detecting signs of electrolyte imbalance, ordering and analyzing lab tests and prescribing appropriate remedies, who is thoughtfully designing and implementing the *nursing* care plan? Will we have time to establish rapport with a family who is experiencing stress and an inability to cope and think logically?"

Of all the issues, the most serious is the cost-cutting climate of today's hospitals. Admittedly, ICU's are still likely to have all-RN staffs. Intensive Care RN/patient ratios are generally appropriate. But even ICU nurses have begun to feel less assured of the continuation of adequate staffing. Already, the least expensive nurses, that is, new graduates from associate degree programs, are increasingly being hired directly from nursing school into ICU, where they cannot practice competently. The better-prepared and experienced nurses, with their own patient load, are expected to supervise these new graduates. It is a difficult situation for both nurses, and it can be a risky one for patients. Often, nurses who take charge of the unit must also do so with no decrease in their own patient assignments. They assume the responsibility for all other patients, handling any number of situations that might arise. Furthermore, ICU nurses are becoming less exempt from the time-consuming non-clinical duties and stacks of paperwork that plague nurses on general medical and surgical units elsewhere in the hospital.

The new problems are not limited to inadequate staffing and non-nursing duties. Hospital-financed continuing education for staff nurses in all areas of practice has dropped drastically in the past twenty years. Furthermore, even in hospitals that boast of expensive, high tech equipment, ICU nurses themselves may be using less visible, older, sometimes unreliable equipment, especially when unit managers have financial incentives to operate on the lowest budget possible. Improperly functioning equipment is not merely a matter of inconvenience for nurses; it can waste precious time in emergencies.

In all areas of the hospital, nurses are struggling against the management mentality of keeping "labor" costs to a minimum. Daily juggling of staff to accommodate cost-cutting is part of the routine. When the patient census is low on one specialty unit, nursing supervisors often have no choice but to send those nurses to understaffed specialty units elsewhere in the hospital. The basis for this practice is management's assumption that a nurse is a nurse, never mind the educational and experience level, specialty, familiarity with the work environment, or familiarity with the patients.

This cost-cutting practice is the result of dire miscalculation in the care of hospital patients. Not only does it place patients in danger; it is actually a very expensive scheme. First, it leaves the unit from which nurses were pulled with inadequate staff should new admissions arrive. Hospital-wide, it creates a perpetual lack of continuity in nursing staff, which is one of the greatest dangers to patients in terms of potential for errors and staff incompetence. It also takes an enormous toll on nurses to practice in unfamiliar environments without the necessary expertise, and it reduces efficiency considerably because unfamiliarity and incompetence can easily double the time required for the nurse to accomplish his or her duties. There are substantial costs to hospitals in increased patient complications, increased lengths of stay, over-time pay for nurses who cannot possibly finish their work in eight hours, on-call pay for nurses and the inevitable patient lawsuits.

The new hospital management's view of nursing care as a series of tasks–changing the dressing, starting the IV fluid, giving the pill, bathing the patient – is part of reason for this practice. Unless nurses are hurrying around at full speed, engaged in tasks, they are not working. In reality, nurses are never at a loss for work to be done, even if it involves time at their desk. No one would suggest that the nurse could leave the unit full of patients, even for a few minutes, simply because there are no tasks to be done at the moment. Nurses are working whether they are moving or not.

Even on Obstetrics, when it occasionally happens that there are more nurses than necessary to care for the number of patients in labor, this "unoccupied" time is important to a nursing staff for many reasons. Among other things, it affords them time to make re-adjustments in the order of the unit, review and rewrite policies, evaluate their handling of previous cases or visit their post-partum patients. Just as importantly, it provides them an opportunity to relax and establish camaraderie so important for any group to work well together, especially when the group works in a very demanding environment. A certain amount of "down time" is essential, and it does not last long. It balances out with those times when nurses have more than they can handle. Such balance is essential in re-grouping and in building and maintaining a strong, effective nursing staff.

We cannot find realistic solutions to the problem of poor quality in our hospitals until we acknowledge that nursing service is at the heart of the issue. The quality of nursing is not only a crucial determinant of the quality of medical practice; very often, nursing *is* medical practice. To target bedside nursing service for quick and easy budget cuts unquestionably places hospital patients in greater danger today than in years past. We must form our strategies on the premise that when nursing practice is at risk, then medical practice is at risk, and patients are at risk. And costs increase.

4

UNCOVERING THE SOURCE OF HOSPITAL MISTAKES

Mistakes and the Hospital's Approach

The National Institute of Medicine has reported that medical errors may cause as many as one hundred thousand deaths annually and more than ten times that amount of injuries or complications. The American Medical Association disputes those numbers, replacing them with five thousand to fifteen thousand deaths. The discrepancy between the two reflects how one defines a medical error. *Both* sets of numbers should give anyone considerable pause before entering such a high-risk facility as a hospital, and they do.

Who is making these errors? Both competent and incompetent persons alike. This immediately tells us that the problem is not merely with individuals; it is in the system.

To refer to these errors as "medical mistakes" is misleading. It creates the impression that only doctors make mistakes or at least, that doctors' mistakes are the ones most worthy of concern. In fact, an array of hospital professionals and non-professionals make both harmless and dangerous mistakes.

It is not an insignificant distinction. Physician errors may be crucial during surgery or wherever physicians are the primary performers of procedures. But on hospital nursing units, most of the mistakes physicians make do not matter. The same is true of hospital pharmacists, dietary workers and others, sometimes even laboratory technicians. By no means are their mistakes inconsequential; it's just that there is almost always a nurse between them and the patient.

When a doctor writes an order on the wrong patient's chart or orders an incorrect medication, the law requires the nurse taking care of the order to question it. The doctor then makes a correction, and that's the end of it. If the hospital pharmacy sends an incorrect medication to the floor, it is the nurse who is held accountable if the medication is administered. Should a lab result not seem logical, the nurse will have the test repeated. Because nurses have the most direct contact with the patient, they are responsible for preventing many of the mistakes of others from reaching that patient. Nurses prevent mistakes more frequently than they make them.

It is not unusual for the nurse to receive a patient's medications from the hospital pharmacy when one or more of the medications is missing. Pharmacies also make errors that are more serious, despite the fact that they are extremely careful and have safeguards in place. For example, a nurse received a syringe containing IV digoxin, a heart medication, instead of the simple heparin flush she had ordered. (A heparin flush is a minute dosage of heparin solution that was used in the past for injection into an IV line to prevent a blood clot from forming within the line and occluding it.) The pharmacy delivered the digoxin in a packet labeled "heparin flush" along with the patient's name, room number, hospital number, date of birth, all the required identifying data. If there had not been a conflicting manufacturer's label on the syringe itself and the nurse had administered the digoxin, it might have been harmful, depending on the patients existing condition. At the very least, the patient's IV line would have become occluded before long, and the nurse would have had to remove it and subject the patient to the uncomfortable procedure of restarting it elsewhere.

Dietary errors occur daily, at virtually every mealtime. Someone delivers a regular diet to a diabetic or a cardiac patient; they inadvertently place milk on the tray of a lactose-intolerant patient or add a straw to the tray marked "no straws" for the patient who has difficulty swallowing. Stroke patients sometimes have an impaired ability to swallow, and they must have all liquids thickened; neglecting to do so can cause the patient to aspirate the liquid. For these reasons, nurses themselves deliver meal trays on some nursing units.

The hospital safety committee, an interdisciplinary committee that meets monthly to review accidents, errors and related statistics in order to recommend preventive policies, generally concern themselves primarily with nursing errors. The reason is simple: by in large, nurses' mistakes are the ones that count. Almost all of the mistakes of others go unreported and therefore unreviewed by the committee because a nurse intervened before these mistakes reached the patient. Because nurses are usually the last links to the patient, nurses' mistakes are thoroughly reported and documented.

When mistakes occur, hospitals have specific procedures for handling them. In the event of a medication error, a patient injury, an omitted treatment or diagnostic test, or any unusual occurrence, the person who makes the error or observes the event writes an incident report. This report is a detailed description of the incident, including where, when and how it happened, who was present, who was involved, and what was done about it. Twenty-four hours later, the patient's nurse at the time adds a follow-up assessment to the report. These reports do not go on the patient's medical record. Once the safety committee reviews the report, the hospital forwards the report to the liability insurance carrier where it is kept on file in case there is a lawsuit.

Naturally, the mistake or incident is also noted on the patient's medical record, but not as an error. For example, if the physician orders 25 mg. of Demerol, and the nurse gives 50 mg. (also a common dose) by mistake, the nurse records that 50 mg. was given. Hospital policy does not permit the nurse to write the word "error" on the patient's chart. The patient's record is accurate, but there is no reference to a mistake. Someone auditing the patient's chart would have to examine it carefully to detect the mistake. In this case, they would have to notice a discrepancy between two different documents: the physician's order sheet and the medication sheet on which the nurse has written the dosage given. Then the auditor could ascertain that 50 mg. was not the prescribed dosage. Usually, no one tells the patient and family about the mistake.

But nurses are consistently reliable about reporting errors to the patient's physician and other appropriate persons within the hospital. They are acutely aware when there is a need for them or the physician to remedy the situation, if possible. If a patient misses a dosage of an antibiotic, for example, the nurse knows that in order for the treatment regimen to be effective, an additional dosage needs to be given. In some cases, the only "remedy," is increased vigilance to observe for signs of problems.

Some hospitals place punitive barriers to the reporting of errors, and in those hospitals, reporting is undoubtedly more limited. But most hospitals do not make an issue of the errors to those who make mistakes – and everyone does – except for the attempts at remedy and the routine procedures for reporting. Naturally, this is not generally the case if the practitioner's mistakes are excessive of have serious consequences for the patient.

Contrary to what the public might think, most mistakes, even medication errors, are relatively harmless. In the event that a patient receives a wrong medication, and it is undetected, the greatest harm is usually that the patient misses the medication he or she is supposed to have rather than the fact that the unnecessary medication itself causes a problem. Still, given the recent revelations of the extent to which harmful and even death-producing mistakes occur, the fact that there are innumerable lesser mistakes is hardly comforting.

Procedures are in place to reduce errors. Such procedures usually consist of checking and rechecking, often by two or even three people, before proceeding. When ordering medications, physicians always specify at least four things: the name of the medication, the dosage, the number of times a day to administer the medication and the route of administration, that is, orally, intravenously, intramuscularly, topically or subcutaneously. Very often, they make other specifications as well. When the pharmacy receives the order, a technician selects the medication, and the pharmacist rechecks it before sending it to the nursing unit. Each nursing unit then has a strict procedure for administering medications and another check system in place to prevent errors. Before giving each medication, the nurse is to note all relevant information to determine that the correct patient receives the correct medication and dosage at the correct time.

The hospital utilizes many check procedures. For example, before administering blood or plasma to a patient, two nurses must check and initial such data as the patient identification, the blood type and the number that identifies the donor's blood as compatible with that of the patient. Laboratory and other technicians who perform diagnostic procedures check patient's identification bracelets and label every specimen. Prior to giving an injection of insulin, two nurses usually check the correct type and dosage. A combination of identifying data must accompany a patient to surgery. Every diagnostic or therapy request form, every sheet on the patient's chart, medication profile or any other document about the patient bears a label with the patient's full name, sex, date of birth, identification number, room number, physician and other data as well.

Some hospitals conduct drills to reduce error and maintain preparedness for emergencies. For drills to be effective, they require qualified instructors who will thoughtfully include a variety of scenarios and meticulously observe and evaluate the staff's performance.

Health professionals routinely employ extreme accuracy in their work. Accuracy is probably more integral a part of the practice of physicians and nurses than any other single element. The realization of even a minor mistake creates a sudden, sinking, terrible feeling within the professional who is responsible.

The story of one nurse illustrates this point. After a corporation purchased the hospital at which she practiced, and it eventually instituted what she found to be impossible working conditions, she not only resigned from that hospital, she also left the profession. She studied hotel management and began working for an expensive, prestigious hotel. The day came when she made her first mistake on the job. The moment she discovered the error, she was visibly shaken and quite upset, but those around her, including the hotel manager, did not find the incident a particular cause for concern. In fact, they were bemused by her "over-reaction." Those with ordinary occupations cannot fathom the seriousness that health professionals ascribe to absolute accuracy.

MISTAKES WAITING TO HAPPEN

So why do hospitals make mistakes? It is easy to speculate about many possible causes because mistakes occur under an innumerable variety of circumstances. But the root of the problem may not be so readily recognized – or acknowledged – by hospitals.

A breakdown in communication is sometimes part of the problem, if not necessarily the root. In one incident of an emergency resuscitation, a child died because the physician ordered intravenous calcium chloride and the nurse instead administered potassium chloride. A miscommunication, yes, but an adequately prepared nurse would not have made the mistake. This incident is not the first in which potassium chloride has been given in error and with dire consequences.

It has been suggested that call-back and "check!" statements, such as those used by pilots, would prevent a breakdown in communication, and sometimes they would. Nurses and physicians often do this already in emergencies, though not with uniformity. But communication is only a preventive factor when there are at least two people. In many emergencies, only one professional — a nurse, a physician, an anesthesiologist or some other — both decides on and administers medications.

Lack of continuing education has also become an issue as surgical techniques and instruments advance more rapidly than practicing surgeons prepare for them. These surgeons may learn directly on their patients with or without an experienced surgeon guiding them. Physicians at times inappropriately use new medications and other treatments that advanced medical knowledge and technology place before them.

Another incident involved an amputation of the wrong leg, which occurred as a result of miscommunication between the person who transported the patient to the operating suite and the person who received the patient:

"The left leg is to be amputated?"

"Right" (meaning "correct").

The right leg was mistakenly prepped for surgery. Both of this patient's legs were in poor condition, which also accounted for the error.

A call-back system would probably not have helped in this situation. Thereafter, this particular hospital instituted the practice of designating the leg that was not to be removed by writing in large print directly on the skin, "WRONG LEG." They thus removed the risk of repeating this particular mistake, though it must be at least a little disconcerting to subsequent pre-operative patients to know that such a precaution is necessary.

Without a doubt, the climate most ripe for mistakes is one in which professionals are working in conditions that diminish quality care in general. On nursing units, mistakes easily occur when there is inadequate staffing, when nurses *lack familiarity* with their patients, when they are distant from patients, and when the responsibility for a myriad of non-nursing tasks diverts their attention. This includes the common practice of pulling nurses from one unit to another where they are not only unfamiliar with patients but also not proficient in the specialized care their patients need. The use of temporary agency nurses and other practices that diminish day to day continuity are very dangerous. All this, coupled with the fatigue and haste under which nurses sometimes must function, considerably increases the risk of mistakes.

An obstetric nurse reported that when there are few patients in their unit at the beginning of the shift, managers frequently pull some of the nurses to work on other floors. Placing such nurses, who may be excellent in their own specialty, in environments that are unfamiliar to them where they do not have the required skills is only part of the risk. In the absence of the regular staff on OB, any number of patients in labor may be admitted; however, the nurses do not return because they are by then obligated elsewhere. When this happens, the OB charge nurse then takes on the time-consuming task of summoning on-call nurses and any others who can be found. Often the nurse is not able to amass an adequate staff; on a weekend, it may be impossible to acquire extra nurses. One OB nurse found herself in charge on the evening shift with a minimum staff when an unusually large number of labor patients were admitted. Ten of those patients delivered. All of her time-consuming attempts to obtain extra staff were to no avail. Her comment at the end of her shift: "Thank God nobody died."

Nurses from other specialties are also sometimes pulled to this OB unit, placing *them* in an unfamiliar situation. A neo-natal nurse, found herself in this very stressful situation. The OB nurses were so busy they had only minutes to orient her.

If these were isolated incidences, it would be understandable, but they are not. This is what many hospitals routinely do to save money, rather than seeking more appropriate means of trimming the budget or utilizing resources. It places patient safety at extreme risk, trusting to sheer luck that the nurses will be able to pull it off. Sometimes the practice is curtailed for a while, once lawsuits begin to rise, but many hospitals continue the same routine on a regular basis.

One nurse describes a recurring dream:

"It varies somewhat, but it is always essentially the same. It is jumbled, confusing and causes enormous anxiety. I am on duty in the hospital. It is terribly busy, and I am far behind. Many of my patients have several IV bags hanging above their beds through which they are getting important medications that require frequent monitoring, but I never check them. I haven't done the necessary treatments, and I can never quite get started with the medications. It's time to give the one o'clocks, but I haven't yet finished the nine o'clocks. New patients arrive, and I can't get to them. The list goes on. My shift is over, it is time to report to the oncoming nurse, and I don't know what I am going to say because I haven't even seen most of my patients."

These kinds of dreams are probably not unusual among nurses. While one might expect such dreams among nurses in military combat conditions or other understandably traumatic service, we should be appalled to hear of them from the nurses in our own community hospitals. The subject of work-related dreams would make a fascinating and revealing nursing research study.

Among these problems with working conditions, the employing of nursing assistants in larger-than-ever numbers is showing a significant impact on the problem of mistakes. Moreover, many of these assistants come from temporary personnel agencies on a day-by-day basis, and they are routinely unfamiliar with their patients or their surroundings. As described previously, non-professionals at the bedside add a new dimension to the issue of hospital mistakes because it is increasingly likely that they, not the nurse, will be the last link to the patient, which removes an important professional safeguard against the mistakes of an array of others.

While nursing units truly need secretarial and other assistance to relieve nurses of non-nursing tasks, patients cannot be assured of safe care if hospitals continue to place nursing assistants at the bedside. Yet, those outside the nursing profession continue to support the hiring of assistants, despite the fact that the only true experts on the matter, that is, nurses themselves, continue to argue that persons who are ill enough to be hospitalized require professional nursing care. If this trend continues – and it appears that it will – it is likely that assistants will soon be doing much more for patients than simple procedures.

One hospital president said, "We need to define the professional nature of nurses more precisely and assign other people to positions where a nurse's professional and scientific background is not essential." This is a typical example of the impudent presumption of those who disregard the misgivings of nurses, making it likely that we can expect more numerous and far more serious mistakes in the future.

This hospital president may feel pressure from the home office, but he is not the one whose heart sinks to the floor at the instant of recognizing a dangerous mistake. He is not the one who must remain outwardly calm while an intolerable level of adrenalin suddenly permeates his body. He is not the one who works with daily fear of having to face a lawsuit (although by virtue of his position, he will be served with the lawsuit) because he directly caused great harm or even the death of another person. He is not the one who will thereafter live with such a burden. He is not the one who reports for duty every day silently praying, "Please don't let me hurt anybody."

While it is not likely that the problem of mistakes will disappear, it can be diminished so drastically that the fear of mistakes would not be a significant worry of hospitalized patients and their families. The difficulty of the problem is not in its complexity; the best solutions are straightforward. It is important to improve safeguards, such as establishing better communication systems, increasing the number and effectiveness of drills, requiring necessary training in new surgical techniques and other treatments, removing barriers to reporting, and utilizing warning signs or labels. But on nursing units, the most effective precautions will be (1) an all-RN staff, (2) primary nursing, (3) appropriate nurse/patient ratio and (4) the elimination of non-nursing responsibilities for nurses.

5

REDUCING CAREGIVERS' RISKS

Many people assume that nurses take better than average care of their health because they are knowledgeable about medicine, nutrition and healthy lifestyle practice. Their career revolves around such things. It is probably true of most other health care professionals that their work has an auspicious relationship to their own health, but it is not necessarily true of nurses. Their health may not be better, or even as good, as that of other professionals.

Naturally, they are at risk of increased exposure to disease. However, such risk is a built-in component of their chosen career, as is maintaining knowledge of recommended precautions. They accept the possibility that they will sometimes become infected, even when they take precautions. They also know that urgent situations sometimes preclude such precautions. Other hospital professionals take these risks as well, though many of them do not have as close or as frequent contact with patients.

Nurses even accept the increased risk of back injuries characteristic of their profession, and minimize their risks by using the body mechanics appropriate for the lifting and bending inherent in their work. Nurses know that back injuries are not easy to avoid, even when good body mechanics are used. The sheer number of times a day a nurse may lift patients, reposition them in their beds or assist them in transferring into or out of bed can cancel out the fact that the nurse may use the correct form each time. Often, the nurse has more than one other patient waiting for her attention with just as pressing a need, if not more so. If the help of another member of the staff is needed for the patient's transfer, extra time has to be taken to locate this person and wait for them to arrive, and sometimes the situation does not allow one to wait.

Whether it is the possibility of sustaining a back injury, contracting an infection, being harmed by a violent patient, or risking their health in any number of ways as they attend patients, nurses are at risk, just as many persons in other fields accept certain risks associated with their work. What is at issue is how these and other risks are *increased* for nurses because of inept, reckless hospital management of their practice.

The case of Diana Morales[4] is an example. She had just completed a twelve-hour shift on a specialty unit that necessarily requires frequently assisting patients with lifts and transfers. When she arrived home that evening, no one has dinner waiting for her, and she couldn't have eaten if they had. Her husband has gone for his 3-day-a-week walk. After her shower, she puts on her robe, pours herself a glass of wine and collapses in the huge, soft chair in her den. She attempts to watch television, trying to empty her mind of the tension and her body of the fatigue.

Like many others, the hospital at which she practices is responding to increasing revelations to the public from nurses across the country that cheaply hired nursing assistants are providing the direct care of patients. The public is hearing that this is a dangerous practice, that assistants are not directly supervised, and that hospital care is becoming more risky. Since hospitals wish to continue this practice, one way in which they attempt to confront the accusations – and perhaps keep their nurses in line – is to pressure nurses to work more directly with the assistants. Besides, assistants work better and more happily if nurses work along with them. But this approach only adds to nurses' burdens. In fact, given the amount of time the assistants can require from the nurse, one sometimes wonders who is the assistant.

---

4. a pseudonym

During her twelve-hour shift, Morales administered treatments and medications for her nine or ten patients, transferred patients, met therapy schedules, processed physicians' orders, answered telephones and performed innumerable other nursing and non-nursing tasks, all the while, she also tried to work alongside the nursing assistants.

Now at home, her mind is too heavy with the worries of the day to watch television. She strolls outside, hurting, picks and tosses a few withered flowers as she tries to soak in the refreshing air in her garden. That night, she gets into bed, relaxes for awhile on her back, then attempts to turn onto her side. To her surprise, she suddenly cries out in excruciating pain. She cannot turn right or left or sit up again in the bed. Only after about four or five hours resting flat on her back is she finally able to change her position without severe pain. At some point during that day, or more likely, gradually over the course of the day, although she used proper technique each time she lifted or transferred a patient, she injured her back. For a long time to come, even slight stress on her back, if sustained for more than a short time, such as during the cooking of a meal, will bring on the painful and debilitating symptoms again.

Despite the fact that back injuries are common, sometimes even causing the nurse to give up her career, most nurses are never compensated for these injuries. One reason is that nurses wrongfully assume (and are led to believe) that because they usually cannot pinpoint the specific incident that caused the injury or because they did not report or complain of the injury while they were on duty, they have no case. Another reason is that nurses seldom attempt to sue their employer for any reason, which is amazing.

But in the end, it is probably not the risk of back injury, infection or bodily harm that poses the greatest health risks in the nursing profession. The greatest health threat to nurses is more likely to be job stress brought on by the inability to practice their profession with a sense of accomplishment and gratification. Moreover, in today's poor practice environment, nurses justifiably carry around with them the apprehension that they will make the big mistake, make the wrong decision or misjudge a priority, neglecting something that turns out to have been all too important.

One nurse said, "In years past, I said a silent prayer each day before I went on duty that God would use me to help patients through their illness. I expressed gratitude for the honor of serving others. Now, every time I get off that elevator and walk toward my floor, my prayers are not nearly so concerned with such luxuries; they are much more self-protective." Daily worry is part of the routine.

There can be little doubt that nurses suffer any number of physical illness manifestations of stressful working conditions. These conditions are often at the root of dysfunctions in their personal relationships as well. Such problems are common when difficulties and frustrations at work seem beyond one's control, and they are understandably magnified when that work carries the emotional burden of caring for the sick and injured, as it does for nurses.

A profession that undertakes the health and well-being of others needs to assess the health of it's own members. There are hardly more important issues on which researchers and nursing leaders could focus than the avoidable risks to nurses' health and approaches to reduce these risks. Affirming the premise that their patients' well-being is bound to their own, as it most assuredly is, is reason in itself for placing a high priority on nurses' health. Even within a profession where there is disagreement on any number of other issues, this issue is surely one of those on which nurses could unite and speak loudly with a collective voice.

6

RESTORING NURSING LEADERSHIP

A SINISTER TACTIC

Alice Macmillan[5] had been on duty since six forty-five AM. She was immersed in the morning's activity when the unit coordinator (head nurse) arrived on the floor at nine.

Today, the unit coordinator, with the most casual of approaches, asks Macmillan if she will come by the office for her (required yearly) evaluation at ten o'clock, implying that the matter is routine and will be dispensed with easily and quickly. The coordinator affably accompanies the request with an apology for not getting to it sooner, but she does "have time to do some of them today."

Taking on-duty nurses from their patients for meetings or other reasons was once a more serious and less frequently allowed event than it has now become. For that matter, such a question today may well be unaccompanied by inquiry about how the nurse's absence will interrupt or otherwise affect patient care. At best, something may be mentioned about asking another staff member to "look out for" the patients of the nurse who will not be available, with the implication that responsibility for one's patients is not a serious matter and that "looking out for" is sufficient.

---

5. a pseudonum

Preoccupied with her work, Macmillan has given little thought to evaluations. Now, she recalls that it is that time of year. Mentally, she begins to re-arrange her patients' care so that she can accommodate the head nurse.

It is a common scenario, but it may well be cause for any nurse practicing today to stop, think and beware. The more nonchalant or off-hand manner in which the unit coordinator approaches the nurse about the evaluation, the more cautious one should be. Such an approach often signals an ambush. That is, the evaluation is going to be negative, and the staff nurse is going to be caught off-guard.

Managers should know that the score one is given in a formal evaluation should never come as a surprise. In any work setting, strengths are to be regularly acknowledged and supported in employees, and unacceptable deficiencies should be dealt with as they occur, not saved for annual evaluations.

Still, even managers who know better often do not operate this way. It is one of the frequently observed phenomena in today's managers that, even when they have ample benefit of hospital-financed management training, often at exclusive resorts, they still use obsolete methods.

Some of the difficulty lies in the fact that being a manager of people necessarily means being a leader, and being a good leader requires personal attributes that are not easily taught by academic institutions. The amount of talent, courage and character one possesses may well bear little relationship to the amount of training or formal education. The difficulty can also be that managers simply do not apply what they learn.

Nursing evaluations may be handled badly for any number of reasons. Sometimes the manager truly doesn't know any better. Sometimes they do not have the courage or the work ethic that good leadership requires. Sometimes they are under too much pressure to provide good leadership or to give enough thought to every aspect of their work, although they might be meticulous in other areas.

But the unit coordinator and the non-nurse department director will handle the Macmillan evaluation very skillfully. The problem in this case is that they will use the evaluation for a purpose other than that for which it was designed. Eventually, Macmillan will be replaced with one who has less experience and less academic preparation, attributes usually accompanied by lower salary expectations and less likelihood to recognize and protest poor working conditions and poor quality patient care.

Nursing evaluations increasingly seem to have little to do with quality of practice, as long as a minimum standard is met. Nurses may sit through an entire evaluation in which the evaluator barely brings up the subject of how well they care for their patients. In fact, the nurse may well exit the evaluator's office with a puzzled expression, attempting to recall whether they discussed the subject at all. Unless their patient care is blatantly negligent, dangerous or in some way an embarrassment, its quality often appears to make little difference in the evaluation. Regardless of where the nurse's level of professional practice falls within the range from merely acceptable to highly superior, it is briefly noted as "standard." The real issues proceed from there.

Many nurses have come to believe that what matters to hospitals is that nurses enable hospitals to be paid, to meet accrediting agency standards and to protect against lawsuits. Nurses must document what the agency wants to see, and their practice has to be such that it promotes the shortest length of stay (not necessarily the healing) of patients because shorter stays are less draining of the hospital's resources. They must also document all chargeable services and supplies. Today, as they write their notes on the patients' charts, what is often foremost on their minds is not necessarily the keeping of accurate patient records to ensure competent care but documenting to forestall legal challenges.

How cheaply the staff nurses will work is also an issue. Not only must nurses be willing to accept a minimal salary but also they must cooperate in allowing the unit to operate with a minimum number of nurses on the staff. This cooperation comes in the form of a willingness to do the work of more than one person and to come in at the last minute when there is a shortage of "help." Working twelve-hour shifts, while not in the best interest of the patient *or* the nurse, is also better for a manager who then has fewer shifts to schedule and fewer nurses earning benefits.

In print, nursing evaluation forms may read like true evaluations of professional nursing practice, and sometimes they are. Others are often lengthy and complicated. Numerical values or checks appear on a long list of criteria. It appears that quality is the focus, but in the end, the evaluations are subjective exercises by nurse managers who may rarely observe the nurses' work, use grapevine information and use the evaluations to whatever end they choose within their scope of power. The evaluation is often simply a measure of how well the nurse fits into a system of functional nursing operated at the lowest possible cost.

In Macmillan's evaluation, the quality of her nursing practice, such as it is within the task-oriented framework of this nursing unit, is not at issue. Individual weaknesses, present in everyone, have been noted and quietly stored, not so much for the annual evaluation, but for the time when it is expedient to make something of them. The manager will also imply, and Macmillan may even become convinced, that her work is not good enough, that co-workers and peers may not like or appreciate her, or that she must carry a heavier workload than she realistically can. The objective is either to bring her into line or replace her with someone more "cooperative" – and less expensive – and it has nothing to do with how well she cares for her patients or with her accuracy, reliability, honesty, professionalism or other criteria of quality work.

While Macmillan's experience should be an isolated, worst-case scenario, more and more nurses are experiencing it. It represents a cynical and fraudulent management tactic, harmful to the emotional and probably physical health of a very large professional group, and it generally works. It is the means to an end, that is, to operate on as scarce a budget as possible, which enables managers to receive bonuses and/or keep their jobs. A few years later, the evaluator in this particular case was also the recipient of treatment similar to that she had doled out to Macmillan and others.

In reality, patient issues should form the basis of evaluations of the work of professional nurses, and most hospitals should use a standard evaluation form. Naturally, other factors may be also taken into account: accurate documentation, reliable work attendance, honesty and so forth. But the criteria should be objective, and anyone evaluating a nurse using this form should produce very nearly the same result. Professional peers, that is, nurses practicing at the bedside, should devise the form. When such a method is used, a hospital manager who chooses to coax higher-paid, more professionally astute nurses into either knuckling under or leaving will have to find means of doing so other than falsifying an evaluation of their professional practice.

The drive in recent decades to turn the public's health care into a lucrative business has lent itself to the taking on of sinister qualities in hospital nursing management. It has nurtured self-preservation and greed in a relatively new and barren management class, the devastating effects of which are directly felt among the general nursing staff, including nursing secretaries and assistants. It inevitably wastes their energy on self-preservation and promotes a certain treachery among them in their relationships with each other.

EFFECTIVE NURSE MANAGERS, AND THE LACK THEREOF

There are *many* excellent head nurses. Yet, far too many of them do not remain head nurses for very long because of persistently burdensome pressure that places their professional values in conflict with the demands of their management positions. The unit coordinator's position can be extremely difficult for one who stubbornly remains patient-centered.

Part of the evidence of this is in the fact that these lower-level management positions in nursing are often hard to fill, though not because the hospital's qualification requirements are excessive. Indeed, during the search for a head nurse, the qualifications are sometimes lowered because the most qualified staff nurses do not want the job. When the head nurse position comes open, it can be impossible to find a nurse on staff who will take it. This is in spite of the fact that it is a promotion for which the salary distinction today is greater than in the past, the hours are decidedly better, and there may be an opportunity for bonuses.

Sometimes department directors coerce nurses into taking the position. Sometimes nurses forfeit their jobs because they will not be coerced. Nurses who take the position often do so for the wrong reasons, and they are not always those who have the desired leadership approach.

Nursing management positions above the level of head nurse do not seem nearly so difficult to fill; at least, when they are, it is not for the same reasons. Those who have advanced their nursing education specifically for the purpose of promotion often hold nurse executive positions, and they may have little patient-care experience. Some of them have barely practiced nursing at all, and they do not attempt to keep their skills current or to maintain meaningful insight into the realities of nursing by practicing even occasionally. Even experienced nurses find executive positions more acceptable, not only because of higher salaries, but because such positions afford distance from the working conditions that exist on nursing units in the hospital. Upper level nurse managers increasingly obtain their advanced degrees, not in nursing, but in business, and they are often not the advocates for good bedside nursing care they could and should be. For that matter, in today's hospitals, their titles often do not even contain the word "nurse." Many practicing nurses view their managers as having little connection to the concerns of the bedside nurse.

Another influence on the effectiveness of nurse managers is that they often must answer to a CEO who does not understand what they're in business to do. The CEO does not understand healing, nor does he or she understand the mindsets of the professionals responsible for healing. CEO's themselves are in a survival mode, which can render them even less willing to listen to their managers' opinions or suggestions for new approaches. This makes it seem that the managers have no choices. Eventually, a nursing manager may no longer respond with anything other than "yes," ceasing to be an advocate for the patient.

It is easy for both nurse managers and executives to get lost in the maze of the everyday issues they face, so distant from the bedside. If there are also financial incentives offered to those who find fast and easy ways to cut costs (and threats to job security for those who do not), then the managers' efforts are likely to focus on cost-cutting rather than establishing frameworks for excellent nursing care of patients.

A MISPLACED MISSION

Practicing nurses are often not aware of the pressures on managers. Staff nurses are immersed in their responsibility for their patients, and they are aware of how their patients are deprived of quality in their bedside care. It is easy for them to perceive this deprivation as attributable to a health care system deluged with greed and buried in excessive management and mismanagement. The difficulty for them is that too many hospitals, whether they are owned by corporations or whether they are among the community hospitals who breathlessly formed alliances in order to compete, have lost sight of their purpose.

Practicing nurses listen to the positive spins of hospital managers, but their own realities are constantly before them. They read the lofty mission statements posted on their unit. They hear the rhetoric about their caring hospital and dedicated staff. Many of them even deny the realities of what they experience (and frequently discuss among themselves) because they would like to be part of something excellent. Yet, they know that today their acutely-ill patient has barely seen anyone except a busy nursing assistant and other occasional hospital persons who stop in to perform their individual, unrelated tasks. Nurses experience the uneasiness of their skepticism about whether the assistant down the hall changing Mr. Jones' dressing or catheterizing Mrs. Clark is using sterile technique. Infections may not show up for several days, so there is no immediate consequence of poor technique. Possible consequence down the road often takes a back seat to the issues at hand. Complications are often not attributable to a specific person. No one staff member is likely to be held accountable. As nurses hurry about their work, they are very much aware of the elderly patient sitting alone at length, staring into the room or the hall, having no one to whom they can express their fears and no one's company to reassure them that they are respected and cared for. The nurse may speak kindly as she goes by, but she only sees to the patient's medications and medical treatments, basic care and safety (it is hoped). Nurses continue to accept such stressful practice, short-changing their patients, because they do not know how to fit into the hospital environment otherwise.

Even when nurses find themselves with free time, they are not always likely to fill that time with patient-centered activity. Granted, they may need the break, but the root of their inertia is probably their perception that even the wise use of occasional free time will not compensate for a poor system.

ADVOCATES FOR THE PATIENT

Bedside nurses are known for their patient advocacy. They often refer to themselves as the patient's best advocate, and they may be right. When a patient's pain medication is not sufficient or appropriate, when patients become overwhelmed with tests and procedures, and in many other situations, it is often the nurse who either makes the changes or takes the patient's case to the physician or other necessary persons. But advocating for the patient cannot be limited to nurses' efforts on behalf of individuals.

Nurse managers, despite the obstacles they face and the pressures under which they manage, must be advocates for all the patients on their units.

They must not lose sight of the fact that they are, first and foremost, nurses. If their professional values are solid, their managerial choices are simple. Both they and bedside nurses will recognize those times when they must say, "I am sorry. This is unacceptable to me." Rather than resigning and moving on to another hospital (nurses are notorious for lateral career moves, where they are only encounter the same problems), they will first ask themselves and their colleagues, "How could better care be delivered? How could *management* influence outcomes?" They will conduct research on their own units, take the initiative to experiment, find the best avenues of care, negotiate with those in higher level management positions, and advocate for what they need.

Standing one's professional ground does not require a hostile approach in order to work with higher management. It may require simply saying, "I understand what a difficult time this is for the hospital. I believe there are three or four approaches we could take to have better care and better outcomes. If the patient gets well faster, you make more money."

Such simple courage and initiative in nurse managers may unveil those qualities in others, both bedside staff and CEO's. Managers may find that their CEO fully understands that one improves their financial position, not by operating cheaper, but by operating better. CEO's may find it very refreshing to be confronted with feasible, well-thought-out and well-presented solutions rather than plagued with more problems. Even when there is only the likelihood of long-term, rather than short-term results, the CEO may allow managers to select one unit in which to facilitate experimentation of how to achieve a better outcome for both the patient and the bottom line. Professional convictions of nurses and physicians are admirable qualities that most CEO's would like to reconcile with the hospital's financial goals if they could find a way. It is well worth the attempt.

A noble challenge awaits hospital leaders with talent, courage, conviction and the willingness to work hard. Both executives and professionals, from their different perspectives, must educate themselves, not just about how to cut costs, but about the *superior economy of good care.*

7

EDUCATING NURSES
WHO WILL PRACTICE
THE WAY THEY ARE TAUGHT

THE THEORY/PRACTICE GAP

"Why don't you teach?"

The suggestion is very familiar to nurses who complain of hospital working conditions. This time the respondent is a young head nurse within whom the rumblings of discontent have reached a boiling point. Recognizing the suggestion as hardly a solution to the real problem, she retorted with a flatly honest response: "Because I could not teach in good conscience!"

The truth is, however, that the suggestion betrays the reason many nursing teachers teach. The occasionally accurate adage, "Them that can, does, and them that can't, teach" may be more correctly stated of nursing as, "them that wish to distance themselves from hospital practice, teach."

The severe compromise of professional practice in many hospitals, which precludes a gratifying nursing career, forces many of the best and the brightest away. A significant number of nursing educators comes from this group of casualties.

As educators, they will be able to do much better work. Although educators experience their own frustrations, their environment is less stressful that that of the hospital where they may deal with life and death situations

91

amid conditions that compromise their ability to do so. They will generally have appropriate assignments of students and will surely have a better work schedule with weekends, holidays, evenings and nights off. No one will be calling at the last minute to ask them to report for duty. They will not be reporting errors or filling out incident reports on a regular basis. They will not be embarrassed by the environment or the quality of their work.

Still, in the end, even nursing educators, no matter how removed they are from hospital practice, cannot remove themselves from an uncomfortable and ever-present realization. That is, much of the professional expertise they are instilling in their students may be abandoned once those students graduate and become part of a hospital staff.

In no other field is the gap between theory and practice more extreme than it is in nursing. From the day they are hired, graduate nurses begin adapting and compromising their practice, a process about which they had received some warning but no real preparation. They know how to practice professional nursing, but when they persist in trying to do so in the hospital working environment, life may become very difficult. The nurse who refuses to compromise good practice may face more stress than he or she is prepared to deal with.

In the end, for those who continue to practice nursing, career patterns over the years are likely to be characterized by a series of lateral moves to various work settings within the hospital or to other hospitals as the nurse hopes for, but seldom finds, a better situation somewhere.

Traditionally, there has been a great divide between many hospital nurses and nurse educators. Hospital nurses have scoffed at educators because what students in the clinical setting are doing bears little resemblance to what the staff nurses are doing. At the same time, clinical instructors privately tell their students not to emulate the practice of the nurses on the unit. The nursing practice portrayed in journal articles by educators has often left their hospital nurse readers wondering if they were all talking about the same profession!

A conversation with the Dean of Nursing uncovers a remarkable perspective.

The question is posed, "Who is the nurse you most admire?"

The Dean named an accomplished nursing education colleague who conducted a significant research project. She considered this person outstanding, and no doubt, she was.

The questioner could not resist re-phrasing the question, "Who is the nurse you would most like to take care of you if you get sick?"

"Oh!" Having acquired a previously overlooked interpretation of the question, she then gave the matter more thought. Finally, she said, "That would be..." This time the answer was someone with different qualities.

To practicing nurses, this would seem to be an unfortunate scenario, especially so because it reflected a school of nursing attitude from the top. But most nurses would not have been surprised by it. Within the profession, direct patient care would not seem to be the most admired area of practice, although logically, it should be, just as it is for practicing physicians.

But in truth, the Dean's initial remarks, although they were off-hand and therefore, presumably most telling, may not have reflected the object of her admiration as accurately as it appeared. As she answered the revised question, her change of countenance and her facial expression actually revealed a deeper and more genuine appreciation for the practicing nurse. With visible crescendo of sincerity and admiration, she carefully searched her thoughts to describe the competence and compassion of one who possessed the gift of excellence in the art and science of nursing care.

To their considerable credit, educators have *thus far* maintained a high standard for nursing theory despite the paucity of acceptable role models for nursing students in the hospital environment. For some years now, they have also worked with hospital nurses in an attempt to ease new graduates into the hospital role by having senior students practice for several weeks alongside a hospital staff nurse preceptor.

It is a worthwhile effort to address the issue; student nurses, like other professionals, should complete such an internship. But with nursing, it still does not get to the root of the problem. Hospital nurses who serve as preceptors for these students speak freely of witnessing the students' expressions of being overwhelmed. In the end, precepting may be an approach that merely accustoms students to falling in line with a money-centered industry.

Today's nursing education must confront the disparity between theory and practice with more than preceptor programs. They must also teach their students that the disparity between theory and practice is the most important issue facing their profession. In clinical teaching, that is, the teaching that takes place in the hospital, educators must acknowledge every example of less-than-professional practice the student witnesses, not just as an object of contempt, but as a focus for instruction. The simple don't-model-yourselves-after-the-nurses-on-the-unit approach has never worked, at least, not after graduation. Instead, hospital-created deficit in nursing care quality must be fully acknowledged at every turn as the patient care problem – and growing crisis – that it is. Nursing schools must teach their students the source of the problem and help them discover appropriate ways to address it, both in their own work settings and in hospital nursing on a national level. Equipping students to recognize poor management and it's effect on their practice and giving them the educational tools to deal with it squarely rather than accepting it as "reality" should be part of the core curriculum. Students must know their strengths, the noble history of genuine altruism in their profession and the inextricable bond between the well-being of their profession and the well-being of their patients. Those who devise the state licensing exam should find these issues of sufficient importance to include them.

It will do little good for students to learn professional nursing process if they are also receive a subtle message that mere task-oriented nursing is inevitable (and apparently acceptable) in their future work settings. When that is the case, they are simply destined to join the ranks of others who practice with persistent guilt and unmet expectations, dreading their work and stumbling through their careers the best they can. In the end, they may abandon the career for which they worked so hard, joining the *hundreds of thousands* of non-practicing nurses. All the while, the ever-more-plentiful movers and shakers in today's money-centered health care industry will continue to mold the nursing profession completely to their liking.

RECONCILING PREMISE WITH PROGRAM

There is another issue difficult to reconcile with nursing theory. Although students may earn a master's or a doctoral degree in nursing, the basic education required to become an RN is one of two levels: an associate or a baccalaureate degree. (There are still a few three-year hospital schools.) This division has a precarious compatibility with an important premise of nursing.

In theory, it goes like this: the associate degree nurses are the "technical" nurses. They practice under the supervision of and according to procedures established by baccalaureate degree (professional) nurses. The focus of technical nurses is primarily on tasks, while professional nurses plan the patient's care, make critical judgments, engage in problem-solving and ethical reasoning, and provide leadership.

Much nursing research has focused on the differences between these two groups – their socioeconomic backgrounds, SAT scores and the roles for which they are best suited. It examines their ability to communicate effectively, solve problems, be self-directed, make sound judgments and provide competent clinical leadership. This research concludes that there are indeed distinctions; nursing schools are educating the two groups appropriately according to the stated differences between technical and professional nurse.

In actual hospital practice, however, it often goes like this: a nurse is a nurse. In most hospitals, one seldom, if ever, hears reference to the distinction between a technical and professional nurse. Baccalaureate nurses are often, though not always, likely to receive preferences for promotion, which usually means being removed from direct care of patients, but hospitals hire both technical and professional nurses for about the same salaries and the same roles. Technical nurses become head nurses and supervisors. They serve on committees and write care plans. They problem-solve, engage in critical thinking and ethical reasoning and perform any of the clinical procedures performed by professional nurses. Patients, physicians and others in the hospital rarely know whether there is any difference in their educational or practice level.

There is more than a theory/practice gap at issue here. Put aside the very significant fact that, theoretically at least, the best nurse is not the one taking direct care of the patient. What is also at issue in this two-level approach to nursing education is that it has a precarious compatibility with one of the essential principles to which nursing subscribes.

Every nurse who has ever taken care of a patient knows that bathing the patient, feeding the patient, changing a dressing, assisting with a bedpan and any number of so-called routine, repetitive, judgment-free tasks provide important opportunities for observing and healing the patient. It is one of the fundamental and unquestionably valid principles taught in nursing school. To a nurse, no patient need is too lowly. (This concept is often obscure to nursing assistants who sometimes think of their tasks as demeaning.) Nurses do not define services rendered to any patient as lowly, lofty, repetitive or in any other way except according to how those services contribute to or hinder the patient's best care. It is an integral part of the mindset of nursing. It is, in fact, one of the most distinguishing qualities of the nursing profession, as it should be.

There is also no such thing as a technical task, at least not at the bedside, and "technical nurse" is a contradiction of terms. The title "practical nurse," long used for those with a one-year period of training, is far more acceptable in terms of both meaning and connotation.

What happens at the patient's bedside is part of a total interaction between the patient and the nurse, and it always influences in some way that patient's recovery or sense of well-being. Procedures and the manner in which they are performed, the observations and judgments made, the revelations incurred, the dialogs between patient and nurse (spoken and unspoken) are all vital elements in the nursing care of the patient. This interaction requires a high level of communication, intellectual skill, sensitivity and compassion, not merely the technical skill to perform a simple (or complex) task.

What created this incongruity in nursing education began about forty years ago, and it was a controversial move. Under pressure to ease the so-called shortage of nurses, nursing leaders "successfully" established two-year collegiate programs for nurses, which replaced the then prevailing three-year (year-round) diploma schools. The "sell" was that nursing students would finally begin to receive college credit for their training.

Even if there had been a true shortage instead of the fact that nurses were leaving hospital practice, other professions would have confronted it by taking advantage of the economic law of supply and demand in order to exercise their clout and improve their position. They would have commanded higher salaries and better working conditions, which would entice new recruits and encourage the return of non-practicing nurses. They would have upgraded their standards to make the profession more attractive to the best high school graduates, and they would have found a means to offer scholarships to these students.

But nurses possess the age-old habit of letting someone else call the shots. There is also their genuinely altruistic mindset, partly misguided at the time, which placed immediate patient needs above their own.

While they were successful at quickly placing more nurses at patients' bedsides, the consequence is that today associate-degree nurses are in the majority. Meanwhile, the problem of nursing shortages continues. Today there is a significant decline in nursing school enrollment and fewer nurses graduating.

Certainly many associate degree nurses are more intelligent, more compassionate and even more professional in behavior than others with more formal education, including physicians. For that matter, associate degree nurses often continue their education. A community college is the source for increasing numbers of students entering four-year colleges in both nursing and medicine, and justifiably so.

Even so, we should not be training registered nurses without providing a thorough ground in both professional character and skill. The basic education for a registered nurse must be a baccalaureate program, which affords students the professional and academic foundation commensurate with the complex care of acutely ill patients rushed through today's hospitals. We cannot merely rely on the possibility that necessary qualities will be found naturally in some graduates, although they sometimes are. Such an educational standard is unrealistic only as long as nurses say it is.

THE PLACE FOR "UNLICENSED ASSISTIVE PERSONNEL"

Another education issue today centers on the training of nursing assistants. Currently, some states require a minimum brief period of training for nursing assistants. Their certification may designate them as level I or level II, according to the number of tasks for which they are approved. Most nurses were happy about this recent upgrading of training because it insured the technical skill training of assistants.

But nurses were deluding themselves again. What has happened since is that hospitals are hiring these nursing assistants in large numbers, at slightly above minimum wage, to replace professional, quality hospital care. While nurses want and need persons who are well trained for secretarial work and other non-nursing responsibilities inherent in running a nursing unit, it is neither safe nor appropriate for minimally-trained assistants to take care of acutely ill, hospitalized patients.

Not only are nurses unhappy with this approach to patient-care, the assistants themselves are not a happy group. They complain of little gratification from their work. They work in the same functional care system that nurses do, according to a hierarchy of tasks, and they perceive their tasks as being at the lower end. The amount of work is often overwhelming. Those who have made mistakes with dire consequences surely regret the day they accepted such responsibility for so little compensation.

In the meantime, while assistants are with patients, nurses often assume other tasks. Although most nursing units employ a daytime and sometimes an evening shift secretary whose services are invaluable, the secretaries do not perform all of the necessary non-patient-care tasks because they have neither the training nor the time. There are too many of these tasks for one secretary, not to mention the fact that managers often occupy nursing secretaries with unrelated work. Nurses then make up the difference in a mountain of non-nursing tasks not otherwise covered on the nursing unit.

If patients are to have competent, professional care in today's hospitals, the only appropriate educational program for nursing assistants must focus, not on patient-care, but on those tasks that keep the patient's professional nurse from the bedside. Tending paperwork, running errands, ordering supplies, checking equipment, assisting with quality assurance audits, answering telephones, posting test results, giving visitors directions, staffing and other tasks too numerous to list can take *as much as 80%* of the nurse's time away from patients. If nursing assistants assumed these duties, they would *truly be* nursing assistants, effective and appreciated both to their own satisfaction and that of nurses.

The struggle against having minimally trained persons taking care of patients has a long history in nursing. Years ago, nurses scored a huge, though rare, victory in their efforts to prevent another compromise in nursing staff education. Again, to alleviate a "nursing shortage", yet another level of nursing was proposed by yet another outside group quite ignorant of the function of nursing but in the end quite willing to listen when nurses asserted their voices *and* suggested other solutions.

It had been proposed that community colleges design an eighteen-month program for Registered Care Technicians, or RCT's. The training was to include a wide range of technical tasks, including the administering of medications. A palliative "there, there" argument was made to nurses that it would relieve them of routine tasks, freeing them for more "professional" functions. Besides, RCT's would surely work under the direction of RN's.

Only because all nurses easily recognized this proposal as such a blatantly obvious blunder did they take an absolutely firm stand against it, forestalling future droves of poorly paid RCT's who no doubt, in time, would seldom work under the direct supervision of professional nurses. It was gratifying to nurses to prevent a scenario that would have had such deleterious effects on patient care. It is not inconceivable that such a move would have opened the door to a future eventually devoid of even the theory of professional nursing, much less the practice.

We have still not closed the door to such a future; in fact, the prospect now looms very close. What has happened since the debate is that hospitals have now hired increasingly large numbers of CNA's (certified nursing assistants). They work even cheaper than RCT's would have worked and have considerably less training. Not only that, a less specific group, UAP's, unlicensed assistive personnel, with little or no training, are now being placed in many departments other than nursing throughout the hospital.

As this has become the norm, nurses dutifully begin the futile struggle to find a route to delegating their practice to others while still maintaining their presence to patients. Never mind the ridiculous idea that the nurse *can* both delegate and be present to patients, which only revives an old burden of nurses that they can be all things to all people. The most important and unfortunate indication from nurses' efforts to cooperate is that, although research continues to confirm that employing nursing assistants lowers the quality of care and reduces patient safety considerably, nurses are once again simply going to adjust and accommodate whoever tells them to do whatever.

Many nurses apparently do not recognize that today's nursing assistants may very easily become tomorrow's RCT's. The idea of upgrading the training of assistants was not only palatable but also welcome, without any thought to possible broader implications for the future of patient care.

Nurses must be alert to any development, however subtle, which will impact the integrity of their profession. Nurses cannot win a battle and then let down their guard. They must consistently determine the best directions for their profession.

Many of the proposals forwarded that would jeopardize professional nursing are not so easily recognized as the RCT proposal. Nursing must acknowledge its history of vulnerability and be exceedingly vigilant. Otherwise, others, however less knowledgeable about the nursing profession, will change that profession according to their own interests.

EDUCATING STUDENTS FOR CHALLENGE

Educators in all fields face a broad range of challenges. Whether in business, law, theology, medicine, education or any number of other careers, curriculums usually must address issues that go beyond their primary focus. Societal changes and trends impact most professions; therefore, most educators understand that they must make their students knowledgeable about these issues. Students must take into account all factors that affect their work. Otherwise, their skills and judgments, even their guiding principles, will not always serve them.

Nursing faces these challenges as well. In the on-going design of nursing curriculum, educators consider the impact of societal and technological changes and other current health care trends. Nursing professors obviously remain informed about evolving issues, and nursing textbooks pay full attention to them. It is an essential part of students' preparation for entry into a "real world" that is more stark in nursing than in many other careers.

Those factors that preclude professional practice comprise the single most important issue facing nursing, today more than ever. Consequently, nursing educators not only face the challenge of teaching the art and the increasingly sophisticated science of nursing, which they do very well, they must also prepare their students to confront a wide range of professional issues.

It is not enough merely to familiarize students with the issues. Nurses who know exactly what they are about will conduct their relationships with hospitals accordingly throughout their careers. If they understand the uniqueness and strength of their professional history, they will not take lightly their role in the evolution of that history.

Other professionals may find it baffling that nurses continue to debate the questions, "Is nursing truly a profession?" or "What is the true definition of nursing?" If nursing schools send out their graduates musing such meek little questions, to which they should have unequivocal answers, it is no wonder the profession has proven so vulnerable. Debate in an academic atmosphere is one thing, but in the "real world" of nursing practice, it is crucial to have solid professional identity. Otherwise, how can nurses be expected to practice confidently?

While it may be healthy for new graduates to lack full confidence in their nursing ability until they have acquired experience and/or further training in their specialty, *it is essential that they are sure of their professional footing from the start.* If students understand that truly heroic efforts were required of nursing leaders in earlier times to bring women of higher education and social status into the profession, will they be likely to endorse less for future nursing schools? If they are certain that the humble bed bath requires a sophisticated balance between strict procedure and fine art and that it is one of the best opportunities for observing and establishing rapport with the patient, will they be so quick to relinquish such procedures to nursing assistants? Will they accept the hierarchy-of-tasks approach? If nurses are certain of their professional identity, their rightful authority in health care and what they require of hospitals, will they passively allow more and more tasks – both those of secretaries and physicians – to be defined by others as nursing functions while their own professional practice disappears? Or will they find their names in the newspaper or on a news show videotape one evening because they passively accepted poor conditions in their facility? Will they feel exploited when they realize that while they compromised their practice and their patients' welfare, they simply enabled others to become wealthy?

Naturally, health care economics is a high priority issue confronting nursing education; the new hospital economy must be an essential part of nursing education. But it must extend beyond learning to stay within the budget. Nurses practicing in hospitals today are aware that they must conserve and charge for supplies, that they must minimize nursing hours, avoiding having even one staff member too many on duty. They understand about meeting third-party reimbursement requirements. Hospitals see to it that staff nurses are properly educated about all those things. What nursing educators must teach their students is how to insure that nursing service receives an appropriate portion of the budget and how to justify economically the systems of nursing and staffing they need.

Hospital nurses also need the benefit of more nursing research relevant to their economic arguments. At present, whenever staff nurses make their needs known, hospital managers need only say that it's not in the budget in order to stop them cold. Nurses must be able to point to research supportive of their economic arguments for primary nursing, all-RN staffs, appropriate RN/patient ratios and the elimination of non-nursing responsibilities. Much of the current research apparently does not enable hospital executives, if they read the findings at all, to make the subsequent correlation to economic advantage, so they are barely impressed. It is probably not too far-fetched to assume that they would require more proof from nurses than they normally would require from other professional groups making requests. The research therefore must be so plentiful and conclusive – *and so publicized* – that it cannot be ignored.

Nurses, like everyone else, must change with the times; they must support the hospital management in its effort to conserve money and resources. But they have a responsibility to the patient—and the hospital—to be alert to compromises in patient care, to assert their observations and their claims, and to participate fully in designing the best systems that hospitals can reasonably be expected to offer. If this is to be the case, nursing schools will need to educate accordingly. They will need research data that proves, in dollars, their arguments for good nursing care. Otherwise, far too little of the patient care education nurses receive will ever benefit their patients.

Educators of nursing students are also in a strategic position to help reverse nurses' history of silence. Teaching students that the silence exists and exposing it repeatedly as a patient-care problem are the first steps. Educators must then teach students to be both assertive and aggressive as a group and as individuals.

Educators must also inform their students that it is essential to become an active member of *one central nursing organization*, no matter how many other organizations they may join. At present, nursing is splintered into many specialty professional organizations—operating room nurses, obstetric nurses, pediatric nurses, cardiovascular intensive care unit nurses and many more. And these are good. These organizations have been one of the best things to happen to nursing because their emphasis is on promoting the best methods of nursing care in their specialty. For that reason, they have been successful in obtaining memberships. Through them, nurses see visions of excellence. Furthermore, in addition to holding memberships in these specialty organizations, many nurses are becoming certified in their specialties. Such certification helps ensure knowledgeable nurses.

On the other hand, the leading umbrella organization for all nurses, regardless of specialty, has not been successful in attracting even a majority of nurses to its membership. *Only about 15% of nurses* belong, hardly enough to give them a strong voice, though the organization has had its accomplishments.

Nurses will site various reasons for not belonging. They may claim that the cost is prohibitive, that the organization has failed to make significant accomplishments, or any number of other reasons. One young director of nurses invited the organization's representative to address the nurses in her facility, yet when they came, the representatives assumed an adversarial posture in relation to the hospital administration right from the start. The director of nursing knew that a partnership relationship was essential. The other nurses did as well.

Professional nurses have distaste for even the appearance of unionizing. They see such activism as antithetical to their altruistic profession. Marching with placards outside the hospital has not usually been their way, although today both doctors and nurses are finding such activity less distasteful than in the past.

It is interesting that nurses are drawn to specialty organizations yet avoid an umbrella organization. Nurses obviously take pride in and have enthusiasm for excellence in their work, yet at the same time, they seem to distance themselves from their profession as a whole.

Whatever the reasons nurses have not united in a central organization, they must discover those reasons and confront them. Whatever the problems within the organization, there is no choice but to find solutions. Whatever contempt nurses may have for their profession even as they take pride in their work, they must acknowledge the need to value that profession and work for the common good. The numbers of nurses are now at two million, and they cannot afford to continue to relinquish the power those numbers afford.

All nurses know that patient welfare is at stake wherever nurses' professional welfare is at stake. While many other groups may unite in order to advance their own interests, nursing has repeatedly demonstrated its proclivity for placing the needs of patients above it's own. Nurses do not fight for higher pay or shorter working hours but for improvements in patient care. Historically, when nurses unite, patients benefit.

It is not enough for educators to inform students of the professional organizations available to them. Educators must explain the situation better. They must convince students that *without a strong central organization, the nursing profession itself will not be strong.* They must candidly examine with students the reasons for and the consequences of the current neglect. By the time students graduate, they must accept it as a given that belonging to a central organization is essential to their nursing practice. For that matter, in view of the present hospital care crisis, nurses may also need to form cohesive groups with other health care professionals who practice in hospitals.

Most nursing students become hospital staff nurses, at least, at first. Their ability to practice what they are taught will require an educational foundation that prepares them to practice well in the face of overwhelming obstacles. Both research and education are of paramount importance in setting nurses up for failure or promoting their success. If students receive the message that the obstacles are too great for their teachers, then the obstacles are likely to be too great for the students. If the teacher imparts the message, however subtle, that hospital bedside nursing is a low aspiration, it stands to reason that graduates who practice at the bedside will not have the professional self-image necessary to appreciate their value to the patient. They will accept their practice as less than it is and on someone else's terms. They may observe other professionals in the hospital confidently performing their jobs well, but nurses themselves will quietly and passively accept that their work will not have the same quality. If they remain in the profession at all, they will leave bedside nursing for any other area of nursing they can – teaching, management, office practice, whatever, as well as any number of non-practice areas within the hospital. They will abandon, if only in spirit, what is the most needed, the most challenging and the most rewarding area of nursing: providing professional nursing care for patients.

According to one nursing leader, "There has to be a place where there are still nurses who come out of nursing school with some idealism and who understand that they then have power and authority to make a difference." Educators, in partnership with practicing nurses, must get to the heart of the matter and devise realistic and authoritative approaches to the theory/practice gap. Such preparation will take much more than a preceptor program simply designed to ease the transition.

Nursing is fortunate to have a role model par excellence. Florence Nightingale lived in an environment in which women supposedly had no way to make change occur. In the struggle to reach her goals, she faced formidable hostility and aggression from those in more powerful positions. Today her legacy is not only the thousands of lives she saved and the gigantic leap in hospital care for which she is responsible, but also the example she clearly left for nurses who must overcome very difficult obstacles.

Following the Nightingale model has not only sustained some nurses but also enabled them to thrive and excel. Of Florence Nightingale, one nurse/CEO says, "She was possessed, or at least, passionate. And passion and obsession can take you just about anywhere, no matter what the obstacles are. When we are talking about the health of a nation, we must be passionate and obsessive about it, and if we are, our sheer numbers and our placement in the process of health care delivery would bring about the change we seek."

8

RECONSIDERING PROFESSIONAL UNIFORMS

A BYGONE PROPRIETY

Nursing students listen with mild incredulity to those who describe the student uniform of thirty-five years ago. The hospital laundry washed – and starched–the dress and apron. Collars, cuffs and buttons were attached separately. At the front center of the collar, students wore a simple name pin, with only an initial for the first name, that is, Miss D. Jones, S.N., (student nurse). There were no hospital ID badges until years later. A specified number of white bobby pins, placed at specified locations, held in place the heavily starched, mandatory white cap, each school's individual design. The student's academic year was, in effect, her rank, (there were almost no male students then) indicated by thin velvet bands or stripes on the cap.

Also standard were the white hose and shoes, the navy blue wool sweater and the wool cape, navy outside with red wool lining and school initials embroidered in gold thread on its neck band. Students kept their hair either trimmed above the level of the collar or worn up. Pony tails were not allowed. There could be no jewelry, except for a plain wedding band (though only by something akin to an act of Congress could a student be married while in nursing school); rings could harbor germs and scratch patients. For the same reason, students trimmed their fingernails short and wore no nail polish. Students could wear modest make-up but not perfume, as the scent might cause nausea in some patients. Students strictly observed the uniform code, and they did not wear the uniform off-campus.

The nursing school guardians of those rules meant business. Where the uniform was concerned, nurses might as well have been in the military, and in fact, the nursing uniform has its roots in the history of nurses' role in caring for the wounded during wartime. Nurses were the first women to be inducted into the military.

After graduation, a strict uniform code remained in effect, although graduates could purchase various styles of white uniforms – dresses, no pantsuits – from uniform shops. They still wore their cap, school pin and name tag in the ordained manner. They wore white shoes and hose and continued to observe the policy regarding hairstyle, make-up, perfume and jewelry.

The uniform code went hand in hand with expected behavior. Nurses were to maintain a certain demeanor and propriety. For example, as implied by the omission of the first name from name tags, nurses did not call each other by first names when they were on duty, even if they were best friends and out of earshot of patients or other staff members. No one else, patients or physicians, called them by first names. As for their inter-action with patients, this was, in theory, the "empathy, not sympathy," era in nursing. Nursing instructors taught students to keep a professional dis-tance, not to become emotionally involved, so they could "maintain their professional judgment and performance." They were not to date male patients, though such a rule was pushing things a bit too far because occa-sionally, students nurses later married former patients. Still, the rule rein-forced the message that relationships with patients were professional, not social.

Today's Uniform, After a Fashion

Anyone who has been in a hospital in recent years knows that all this is very different from the present-day expected behavior and dress code for nurses. Today, hospital nurses wear almost anything they like, including street clothes. Emergency Room, ICU and OB nurses, among others, usually wear scrubs because they're practical, simple and comfortable. Pediatric nurses often wear scrubs decorated with cartoon characters to please their young patients. Various styles of walking shoes, socks or hose, colored blouses, whatever, are generally worn by nurses today. And of course, no one wears a nursing cap.

Nurses may or may not wear school pins, and jewelry is acceptable. Just about any hairstyle is acceptable, and there are no restrictions regarding make-up or perfume. Hospital ID badges have long replaced simple name tags of "D. Jones, RN," and wearers generally place them anywhere they like as long they are reasonably visible. The ID badge is probably the only item consistently mandatory, though some hospitals are surprisingly lax about that requirement as well. Almost everyone refers to each other by their first name.

The relaxation of uniform standards in the past few decades had some basis in the theory that patients would be more comfortable with the nurse's "less distant" attire. Something closer to everyday wear would ease the cold and often lonely environment of the hospital, especially when patients' hospital stays were longer than they are now. Educators particularly espoused this opinion, and nurses in general accepted it. As a matter of fact, the changes in uniforms coincided with other changes, such as pastel bed linens, papered walls and other departures from the stark physical environment and ether-permeated air of the past.

But there may have been less obvious reasons behind the change in the nurse's uniform. At the same time opinions about the uniform began to change, intensive care units were becoming more widespread in hospitals. Almost overnight, a new nurse emerged, more active, more involved in clinical decisions, with more authority in emergency situations, more spe-cialty-oriented post-graduate training and a stronger collaborative rela-tionship with physicians. Suddenly, hospital nursing had an important new focus. The profession made a giant leap in becoming more directly involved in major clinical decisions. Life and death judgments became an everyday nursing function. As all this happened, some of the profession's former proprieties and rituals, including strict dress codes, assumed less importance. Indeed, a discarding of old rituals and dress codes and the discovery of more substantive practice was a wonderful breath of fresh air.

It was interesting to witness this remarkable change. The new ICU nurses recognized and respected the hospital's best doctors more than ever, and overall, nurse-physician relationships improved immensely with the advent of these units. The submissiveness of nurses now began giving way to a closer, more clinically complementary relationship between nurses and physicians on the patient's behalf.

Most nurses adapted well and did not find their new participation in medical decision-making confusing at all. As this new relationship evolved between the two professions, their respective professional identities remained intact. In fact, the nurses in one ICU posted a sign in the nurses' station just so everyone would know: "not junior physicians but super nurses."

ICU's were a revolution in hospital nursing. In one quantum leap, nursing had changed forever, and the effect was more than the sudden, drastic reduction in patient morbidity and mortality. It elevated the ICU nurse's confidence, revealing greater possibilities of nurses' practice and increasing the gratification they received from their work. And it gradually swept the entire nursing profession.

The point is, as nursing practice changed, professional behavior and uniform attire also changed. What changed about the uniform was that it began to seem more practical to wear very simple clothing, such as the scrub suits that were already worn in surgery and OB. These scrub suits became common, first in ICU's, then in other areas of the hospital. With advances in nursing and better working relationships with physicians in their sights, nursing schools began changing their uniform codes as well. The apron was out-dated first, with its handmaiden connotation; later a few nurses discarded their caps for the same reason (though most just felt that the cap was a nuisance). Gradually, other aspects of the dress code, such as jewelry, nail polish and hairstyles, relaxed also.

All of this was taking place during the additional societal trends of the late 1960's and the 1970's. Simplicity, self-expression and disdain for ritual and materialism became the order of a large segment of the new generation. These trends undoubtedly influenced the current generation of nurses.

There was another less recognized influence on the relaxation of nurses' uniform standards. It was about this time that corporations began widespread buying of community hospitals, and there was rapid change in the business. More money was suddenly available, at least at first, for equipment and training, as well as what appeared at the time to be refreshing, innovative approaches to running the hospital. As this began taking place, there were also increasing numbers of management/clerical persons, consultants and support persons of all descriptions. Whoever they were, they proliferated, all wearing suits and street clothes heretofore much less visible in a hospital setting.

The uniform code, what was left of it, once again became a casualty as nurses found themselves with a broader realm of job possibilities other than direct practice. Even those who continued to practice were now sitting in conferences or meetings of various kinds more than ever before. Amid all this, there was the subtle message that street clothes implied higher status.

Except for the early decision to change to "less distant" attire, educators and nursing leaders passed down no considered opinion recommending a change in the professional nurse's uniform. There was no formal consensus among hospital nurses to change their uniform from what it was to something else. Instead, change was the slowly-occurring result of nurses' attempt to put their patients more at ease in the hospital environment, nurses' wish to remove a servant appearance, nurses' laxity about their uniform standards, a desire for more practical clothing and the intrusion of corporate influence on the profession. Most of the changes in the nursing uniform over the past thirty years or so were not planned; they just happened. And therein lies a problem.

A NEED FOR REASSESSMENT

Today, more than ever, nurses cannot afford to let anything concerning their profession "just happen." And while some may think that the uniform is the least of their professional concerns at this time, that is not necessarily the case. The laxity of standards in today's uniform has fast become just as inappropriate as the strict standards of years ago.

Nurses are now barely distinguishable to patients. Although this may work to the advantage of the images of hospitals that are utilizing so many non-professionals, it hardly works to the patients' advantage.

Nursing assistants often appear to be nurses. This practice produces the illusion of an adequate nursing staff to the public. It is illegal to represent an unlicensed person as a registered nurse, but with the relaxation over recent years of the nurse's uniform requirements, it is easy to obscure the distinction without overt misrepresentation. One may even hear nursing assistants say to patients, "I'm your nurse today." Their tone implies, not that they are lying, but that "nurse" is a general term for whoever takes care of the patient. It is an easy charade with the increasing blend of non-professionals and professionals in nursing. Patients and families often identify assistants as nurses and assume the hospital is well-staffed, even though the "nurses" do not seem very professional to them.

Everyone knows what a nurse in standard uniform looks like. Nursing is one of those professions whose image includes a certain appearance, just as that of a police officer or a priest. In the past, patients and families had the advantage of being able to recognize the nurse instantly simply by the uniform, and that instant recognition served a purpose. It is important to be able to distinguish nurses from others in the hospital.

It does not suffice that nurses merely introduce themselves to patients. For one thing, patients are often under severe stress – emotional, physical or otherwise. They may be distracted or disoriented or barely conscious. For any number of reasons, patients may not be able to comprehend or remember what is said to them. Still, they are likely to recognize the nurse in a traditional uniform before any other person in the hospital. By virtue of their profession, nurses have an instant, built-in rapport with patients, a distinct advantage in caring for the sick.

Just as the uniform itself is instantly recognizable, so is the abbreviation "RN." To many people, it is comprehended as readily as "USA." Simple, clear name pins with only the letters "RN" following the last name may allow even very ill patients to recognize the nurse.

The ID badges currently used in hospitals, on the other hand, are not that clear. They usually bear a small photograph, after a fashion, of the wearer. The wearer's name is followed by any number of abbreviations that are often a mystery even to other professional personnel, much less patients. The badges include a lot of information in a small space, such as the department, the name of the hospital and the name of the corporation. They hang from any one of various locations on the uniform, including the waistband or pants pocket; they may be turned backward or possibly not worn at all. Some hospitals do not strictly enforce their policy about wearing the ID badge, even though the primary purpose of the badge is for hospital security. At any rate, if the patient is to read and understand the name and job title, he or she must be alert, have good eyesight, and not be under too much stress to consider who is who. In effect, the hospital ID badge is hardly the patient's best source of identification of nurses.

Perhaps the theory was correct that the traditional uniform conveyed distance, which did not always work in the best interest of the patient-nurse relationship. Yet, patients have always been more likely to ask questions or discuss their concerns with nurses more than with physicians or anyone else in the hospital. Actually, this may be less true today, despite relaxation of uniform attire, because all too often the nurse is not around long enough and is not as likely to be familiar to the patient. In the absence of primary nursing, the patient may find that there is no one with whom he or she can discuss some concerns, and the uniform itself has had no bearing on this issue at all. If anything, the change from the traditional uniform has reinforced the lack of a real nurse available to the patient because they cannot distinguish the nurse from others.

One could also argue that the supposed distance conveyed by the traditional uniform might even work to the patient's advantage. Much of the contact nurses have with patients is potentially embarrassing for patients, and a professional distance eases such embarrassment. Nurses can still convey caring and concern to a patient, even with the matter-of-fact manner of a professional. A professional nursing uniform, a modest hair style, and other "out-dated" elements of the dress code also may convey dignity and respect to the patient, who in their current predicament, easily finds their dignity vulnerable.

It's easy to understand why many nurses, such as those in ICU, ER or OB prefer the practicality of scrubs suits. But there have also been other reasons for the preference for scrubs. Many persons in any number of departments in the hospital now wear them. They identify the wearer as someone whose function is perhaps a little more sensational – and presumably more important – than that of others, just as street clothes came to suggest higher status during the corporate "takeovers." The problem is that just as a professional uniform or any other aspect of one's appearance conveys certain messages to patients, so do scrubs. Perhaps a subtle message from scrubs is that the wearer is primarily a technical person: "My focus is strictly on your 'important' clinical needs. Look to someone else to be concerned with you as a whole person." Furthermore, some persons who wear scrubs are mistaken for surgeons.

As for the handmaiden connotation, the uniform may have little or nothing to do with that. As ICU nurses proved years ago, the quality of relationships with other professionals has to do with the type and quality of nurses' professional contributions, and little more. Those contributions are most determined by the nurse's individual character, competence, education and working conditions. Many nurses, especially those who practice on general medical-surgical floors, or even in some specialty units now, will tell you that they feel more like handmaidens or something akin to waiters and waitresses today than ever before.

Nurses may not need to re-instate traditional uniforms, caps and all the other features of what was once mandatory dress. But they do need to consider the significance of the professional uniform and its implications for their practice. They need to reassess the role of a professional uniform, its message to patients and families, its function in infection control, and its function in enabling the nurse to fulfill the optimum professional role. Uniform standards need to be taken seriously, regardless of whether they are, in the end, retained or discarded. Whatever the case, it is the nursing profession who should thoughtfully determine those standards. The professional uniform should not be left to the casual needs of the moment, and it should not be a matter of individual hospital policies formed by managers with little insight into or concern for the matter except for that which is related to their own economic goals.

9

ENABLING PUBLIC ACTIVISM

Nurses have neglected the nurturing of a public image. Nurses tend to think only of their rapport with individual patients and in terms of how it affects the patient's recovery and well being. They have not focused on a public image, even as they've gone about their practice, which itself is only partially visible to patients. Consequently, much of the public image of nurses has been created and advanced by others.

Today, hospital nurses find themselves expected to nurture a public image — not their own, but that of the hospital. The hospital requires that nurses, along with all hospital personnel, attend "guest relations" classes, often taught by one of the increasing numbers of hospital PR persons. Nurses go along without objection, even though they may feel that such superficial instructions are useless to them as a professional group, and they express concern that hospitals are increasingly replacing competent professional care of patients with the practice of being friendly to the "customer." As professional practitioners, they are discerners of the difference.

Meanwhile, direct professional contact with the public as patients and family members is the primary means through which nurses' public image is molded. Unfortunately, the quality and frequency of that contact is too often less than it should be. Except in ICU's and some specialty units, the contact nurses have with individual patients and families in hospitals is usually in brief increments during the performance of tasks.

Twenty years ago, such dark-ages nursing care was becoming the practice of the past. The prospects of primary nursing and all-RN staffs were within sight, and some hospitals even featured their primary nursing in advertising. Today, however, what was once welcome progress is reversing, as task-oriented nursing is again becoming the norm, replacing true nursing process in many hospitals. Many of today's associate-degree nurses do not envision anything different. And it is these nurses, along with nursing assistants frequently mistaken for nurses, who are more likely to be in direct contact with patients and families. Baccalaureate degree nurses and those with advanced degrees are found less frequently at the bedside.

The public is likely to regard nurses as persons whose most significant function is carrying out physician-prescribed treatments rather than having a separate, professional relevance to the patient's progress or recovery. Given the growing inability of nurses to provide professional care in today's hospital environment, the current limited educational requirements for registered nurses, the very brief contact, if any, that a professional nurse actually has with the patient, and nurses' tradition of silence, it is only logical that the public should hold such a perception.

Nurses and the environment in which they practice are responsible for this image, but there are other public image problems as well. In television and movies, nurses have been portrayed as everyone from the stern prison-warden type to the gentle, "yes-doctor" handmaiden in television and movies, not to mention the inevitable less-than-articulate, bleached blonde in sexually suggestive dress.

Naturally, the public accepts such characterizations as fantasy, and today, many of the television movie images of nurses are less stereotypical. Besides, many viewers know that hospital-type shows are seldom realistic, even when they are meant to be. Movies are generally for entertainment, not realism. Even those movies that are true works of art do not necessarily depict realism in plots, settings or characters.

Still, repeated images have an impact. Viewers often judge today's hospital shows by how realistic they seem, and when they perceive them as such, the portrayal of the role of nurses takes on added significance. As a matter of fact, currently there is a new and disturbing development with regard to the image of nursing – and doctoring – in television movies, that is, the new sensationalism. If the public assumes that such action-packed images are complete and accurate, then we are in trouble with regard to what young nurse recruits will be looking for. Recently one young nurse, describing in a television interview his excitement about nursing, labeled himself a "trauma junkie." Most of us would prefer to be cared for by a nurse who chose the profession for reasons other than a desire for excitement and sensational hospital drama.

The public image problem for nursing is not only with theater or television movies but also with the news media. Networks today frequently report medical advancements and hire physicians as reporters. Yet, it is not so much what news shows report as it is with what they omit that leaves the public ill-informed about the quality of hospital care in their communities.

The news media has paid little, if any, attention to the fact that major advancements in hospital care, both today and in the past, have taken place as much in nursing service as in medicine or technology. When Coronary Intensive Care Units (CICU's), for example, began opening over thirty years ago, the mortality rate for hospitalized heart attack patients dropped almost instantly by *thirty to forty percent*. To someone with cardiac problems, that tidbit of information would have been of more than passing interest. Yet, not only was the public not made aware of the significance of ICU's, but for some time, many doctors were reluctant to admit it as well. What accounted for the absence of news coverage was undoubtedly the fact that these units did not utilize new technology or medical treatments that had not long been available; they were instead based exclusively on an advanced system of nursing care.

CICU's were more than a leap forward in themselves; it was from them that other advances in medicine and technology emerged. Other kinds of ICU's and specialized units followed, lowering mortality rates even more and improving care immeasurably. New medical treatments quickly began to arise as a result of the knowledge gathered from closer observation of patients. These units also spawned advanced training in community emergency medical services. CPR training is now common among the public, and defibrillators may be found in office buildings, airplanes and many other locations. Consequently, today's mortality rates are significantly lower not only for hospitalized patients but also for patients before they reach the hospital.

Another "medical" advancement almost single-handedly promoted by nurses was the Lamaze method of childbirth. Most obstetricians were initially unconvinced of its value and feasibility. Even doctors who thought the idea had merit would not publicly endorse it in the beginning for fear of jeopardizing their own professional image and consequently, their practice; they instead supported nurses from behind the scenes. Today, Lamaze classes are an integral part of preparation for the birth of a baby, which physicians accept and promote as a matter of course.

Before the Lamaze method became well established, the environment on obstetric units was quite different than it is today. Before Lamaze, hearing labor patients cry out from pain and anxiety were routine, while fathers paced and worried outside. After Lamaze, obstetric units became much calmer places. Patients' pain was better controlled, and the process of childbirth with a father or other supportive person present was a much more positive experience.

Nurses were leaders in patient education in general, again without initial support from many physicians. Some physicians were in outright opposition to patient education. Many were concerned that if they suggested possible medication side effects to patients, patients would naturally anticipate the side effects to the extent that they would think they were experiencing them or would actually experience them. Doctors sometimes gave little information to patients about their illnesses, including diabetes and other chronic diseases about which it is crucial for the patient to be well-informed. At best, they felt that decisions about how much to tell patients fell only within the physician's sphere of authority. Meanwhile, a patient taking a prescribed diuretic could acquire a stomach virus from some source, resulting in vomiting and diarrhea, and become severely dehydrated simply because they did not know to discontinue the diuretic, one of the innumerable problems that may result when poorly-informed patients take medications. It is because of nurses that educating patients about their illnesses and treatments has become an established component of hospital care, required by the accrediting agency and the law. Pharmacists now distribute educational leaflets along with the drugs they dispense. Nurses initiated these and many other such advances in health care.

Still, nursing contributions are comparatively rare subjects of news reports. The problem is that the news media, as excellent as much of their work is, can be decidedly biased, however unintentionally, in their reporting of health care issues. A shortage of nurses is about the only nursing issue that catches the attention of reporters, and even that report is misleading. Adding to the problem is that news shows, unlike movies and other television shows, are taken seriously.

Most of us have come to expect a lot from our free press. We take instant, accurate news for granted. We shudder to think what it would be like to live in a country where there is no such valuable service to the citizenry; therefore, we place minimal constraints on journalists. As some news reporting descends to tabloid quality, we even tolerate being barraged with sensational and increasingly graphic horror stories, though today more of us censor our children's viewing of even major network news – and surely local news – just as we do other programs that are not mindful enough of the young audience. We also accept that one does not report the cat that did not get stuck in the tree, so we accept a one-sidedness in news reporting that would give a stranger to our planet a distorted view of our communities. We acknowledge that the economics of television dictate that even the best of news shows must consider not only what is newsworthy but also what commands interest or what can be designed to command interest. We understand that reporters, like the rest of us, are likely to hold many of the larger society's attitudes, for example, that the higher income a given profession has managed to secure for itself, the more value it holds for the society.

Certainly we are fortunate to receive what may be the greatest quantity and the most in-depth political coverage of any news media in the world. Each government activity and each politician's motive, background and personal life are researched extensively and reported repeatedly. There is a concerted effort by the media to dig deeply and explore beyond obvious facts and events, to provide the public with important information about their government and political system. If any institution should be so scrutinized and reported, surely it is government, with it enormous power over the lives of the people. A free press minimizes the abuse of such power.

We must recognize, however, that today's health care system has also come to hold extreme power over the lives of the people. Its cost has reached unimaginable amounts, impacting the quality of the lives of average persons, sick or well, every day. How many persons live in fear because they are among the approximately forty million currently without medical insurance? How many persons have faced bankruptcy because the medical bills they receive are several times over the cost of their house? How many persons must pay excessive fees for treatment of routine illnesses because they have nowhere else to turn but hospital emergency rooms when the time comes? How many persons, even with insurance, avoid necessary visits to their doctor, because they, and each member of their family, must pay several hundred dollars of an initial deductible amount before their insurance carrier will pay one dime? How many persons, with or without insurance, who live with chronic illnesses or take care of a family member who does, also live with chronic financial worry? How many young families are there in which both parents must work only because they will not otherwise maintain enough health insurance, and place very young children, even infants, in day care in order to do so? The scenarios have become endless. All this is in addition to the tax burden of necessary government health care programs.

The point is, just as the public needs to be well informed about the activities of their government, they also need to be well informed about an immensely powerful health care system. Legislators must be knowledgeable enough to make health care policy decisions. Individuals need information that enables them to make good personal decisions concerning hospital care for themselves and their families. And community leaders must be able to recognize the level of quality in our hospitals.

The high quality of coverage of the events of September 11, 2001 is proof that major newspapers and television networks are capable of doing their job exceptionally well whenever they are determined. They are just as capable of excellent reporting in other areas. As our country has freed them from the constraints of censure, they must also free themselves of the constraints of questionable, even mistaken, perceptions. As they seek out the hidden agendas and the less-than-obvious facts in other areas of reporting, they can bring the same high quality and determination to their reporting of the workings of our health care system (whose function may now include being a first line of defense against our enemies). Yet, if journalists lack meaningful insight into this powerful institution, if they are confused and intimated by its complexity, then they can be sure the public is as well.

By taking the time to acquire a deeper grasp of the situation, journalists can provide an immeasurable service to their viewers and readers. Granted, substantive reporting in health care demands time-consuming, careful research. It requires the same willingness to look beyond the surface that reporting on other important issues requires. It takes thought and talent, not only to discover the issues, but also to report them in such a way that the public listens and understands their consequences. And it requires contacts, not just at top management, but at the direct-patient-care level because in health care that is where the story is. Ask any nurse (and many former patients) and the answer is generally the same: "I could give you an ear full."

Journalists have a crucial role in determining whether we have, or do not have, quality health care. To meet that responsibility, they must grasp the truly substantive issues in health care. They must know that the latest articles in prominent medical journals may not be nearly so germane to the concerns of the public as the systems of nursing care in hospitals. They must know that the issue of physician-assisted suicide is not more important that the less sensational issue of whether or not a professional nurse (and it is most likely to be a nurse, not a physician) is available to assist terminally ill patients and their families. Along with their community hospital's press release of employee of the year, local reporters must also discover the number of nurses in their community who are not practicing solely because of the hospital's working conditions. When reporting the high cost of health care, they must delve into the high cost of mismanagement, incompetence, cowardice or greed.

The power we grant our free press must pay off in returns of insightful health care news coverage on both a community and a national level. This will not happen until journalists, both local and national, sharpen their focus on the nursing profession, not to raise the status of nurses but to reveal the full significance of nurses to our welfare as hospital patients. Not only are nurses essential to the solving of our hospital care problems, but they know so much that they aren't telling.

10

RECONCILING POWER, PROFIT AND SERVICE

THE PROFESSIONAL IMPERATIVE

One hospital executive remarked that selling hospital care is no different from selling food, his point being that since it is acceptable to profit from the sale of one essential item, it is also acceptable to profit from the other using the same sales approach.

Over the past thirty years we have learned more than we ever wanted to know about the management of hospitals. But what we've really learned is what we already knew: that the *primary purpose* of the hospital cannot be monetary. When the product is penicillin, pre-natal care, an emergency tracheotomy tray, or hospital care, then the business enterprise is unique.

Hospital patients are by no means customers in the ordinary sense. It is absurd to assume that an ordinary business transaction is taking place when the one buying is doubled over with a gallbladder full of stones or has a child bleeding from a gunshot wound. To view hospital service as an ordinary commodity, to refer to the sick and injured as mere market share, is not acceptable in a humane society.

We are also re-learning that it is illogical for health care professionals to become hired hands of industries that operate only for profit. Health professionals are distinguished from others by an orientation to service. They focus on theory, research and practice, but their single most distinguishing feature must necessarily be altruism. The most logical arrangement is one in which they themselves are the hirers of accountants, attorneys and business managers, not the reverse. Physicians, nurses, pharmacists, nutritionists, therapists and the other valuable health professionals in the hospital – these are the people we want calling the shots when we are patients. It is hard to imagine that anyone, even the strongest supporters of private enterprise, which most of us are, would prefer to have their hospital care directed by anyone else.

Health care professionals cannot focus only on their work, looking to others for leadership of the industry as a whole. The designing of hospital care systems depends on those who have the knowledge base, the credentials and the licensing that afford them self-regulation and autonomy to function in the public's best interest. They are automatically participants in leadership, both as individual professionals and as part of a professional group.

The nurses on whom hospital patients depend for both care and cure cannot continue to react to ill-informed leadership outside their profession either by accommodating to conditions or by abandoning their profession. They cannot continue, as they traditionally have, to work silently and anonymously, sometimes distancing themselves emotionally from their work, and therefore, their patients. They cannot design nursing education only to accommodate the hospital's economic goals or design preceptor programs for no other reason than to lessen the reality shock for new graduates moving into the work world where their practice will then cease to be professional and become a series of tasks.

They must not settle for a mere semblance of their practice under whatever circumstances presented. They must instead become as vocal or as united as they have to be to promote the care of patients. Struggling day after day to provide a bare professional service to patients is not the struggle that will help their patients in the long run, nor will it help the future of their profession. If they are to live up to the Nightingale legacy, they must operate differently.

Hospital nurses must be more effective in communicating their roles and their strengths to CEO's and to others. They must make it known that the character of nursing service is a strong determinant of the hospital's mortality rate, the length and quality of patient recovery, the frequency of hospital mistakes and the number of lawsuits. It is they who are in the best position to be conservers of resources. They are also the least expensive, yet the most expert, consultants and efficiency analysts when their talents are so used. They require opportunities to experiment and to demonstrate the benefits of their professional ideas, in alignment with sound hospital economics.

If instead nurses willingly allow their profession to be molded according to the interests of short-sighted, ill-informed, non-professionals, especially those who may be in this business *only* to make money, should they not expect it to happen? Should they not expect professional hospital nursing practice to be maintained only as long as it serves that end? Should nurses be surprised when those who are ignorant about their profession, what it requires and what it has to offer, simply view them as "their largest labor force," turning a deaf ear until the budget is trimmed to satisfaction?

It is unfortunate that nurses expend much time and energy bemoaning their lack of power over their practice in hospitals. Given the lamentations that have long arisen from the ranks over this issue, one would think it would at least be a subject for required instruction in nursing schools.

Power is always available; the problem is, it is not well understood, and it often lies dormant. Seizing it is a matter of will and alertness to windows of opportunity. It is inherently available in the professional authority of nurses, but by their silence, they affirm the power of others. As individual professionals, they are automatically empowered to do the right thing, to teach, to direct, to delegate and to serve as role models. They are empowered to challenge any authority that comes between the patient and proper care. Through sheer numbers, united, they could use their collective power to effect positive changes in their hospital practice.

One must remain aware that there are two ways to abuse power. Naturally, one is to use it aggressively to harm or exploit those who are subordinate or weak. But what is probably the most frequent misuse of power is to fail to act or to remain silent when there is a need to be heard.

Nightingale set an example few nurses have followed. Her lesson for us was that power does not have to be delegated; it must be seized. In the Crimea, when more soldiers were dying from infections than battle wounds, she and the other nurses scrubbed clean the vermin-infested barracks that they themselves were given as living quarters. During the night, they then moved wounded soldiers into this area, cleansed their wounds and reduced the death rate by fifty percent! All the while, they endured the antagonism of a hostile chief surgeon who refused even to utilize the anesthetic Nightingale had brought for amputations. Eventually, she demonstrated the merits of her case statistically and sent a letter to the surgeon's superior officer *on behalf of the soldiers, her country and her profession.* The chief surgeon was removed from his post.

Nightingale's principles drove her actions. Neither title nor position of those "in power" inhibited her. At a time when women supposedly had no way to bring about change, she did not accept that women or nurses were powerless. She did not wait for permission to act. When persuasion alone failed, she developed a strategy, and she used imagination. Nightingale has thus left a clear message for each individual nurse at the bedside today.

The views of today's hospital managers may seem ill-informed and short-sighted to nurses, both from a patient care and a business perspective. But it is nurses who are unrealistic if they continue wasting time waiting for others to see the light. Nurses must realize they themselves bear the responsibility for accepting the conditions of inappropriate patient assignments and a myriad of non-nursing tasks that cause them to short-change their patients. It is they who allow their contributions and the enormous advances nurses have created in hospital care to go unknown, unappreciated even within their own profession.

Although nurses comprise a distinct profession, authorized to define nursing practice and determine their own standards, they fail to do so. They wait for someone to allow them to practice what they were taught, for some entity outside themselves to give them permission to take their place as an autonomous, authoritative professional group. All the while, the "entity" simply molds them and uses them to whatever end meets its own interests. This great sin of omission, which characterizes the nursing profession, constitutes nothing short of a silent malpractice robbing the public of the hospital care it is supposed to be getting.

The plight of nursing is their own failure and their own responsibility. Whatever decisions nurses do not make for themselves, others will make for them. When practice does not measure up, it is the practitioner who is culpable. Only when they understand and accept this unequivocally, taking full responsibility for their own practice, will they be able to deal effectively with this tired old issue, which has today become an urgent issue.

When nurses – or physicians – tell you that they are required to practice according to a lower standard, they are wrong. What is true is that they agree to practice this way. When they say that they have lost autonomy, what they really mean is they have relinquished it.

Nurses cannot expect others to have insight into what their profession is about unless nurses tell them. It is not realistic to blame others because *their* practice does not measure up to what they were taught in nursing school. It has not worked to leave this to nurse educators or nurse managers, or any other nursing "leaders" who themselves may have become distant from the practice of their profession. It is practicing nurses who must expect nothing less than a work environment that enables them to fulfill their duties to their patients as they were meant to be fulfilled. When it comes to excellence in their practice, bedside nurses must get the picture: the buck stops with them.

If nurses do not attempt, through professional cohesiveness, determination, persistence, vigilance and wise strategy, to reverse some of the unfortunate current hospital nursing care trends, no one else will. They can only do so by operating in the full spirit of Nightingale reform. If risks must be taken, so be it. Transformed careers must be expected. Nurses cannot continue merely fitting into the plans of others, maintaining a tradition of silence, thus, condoning unsafe, assembly-line care for their patients.

The full acceptance of this responsibility is within their scope if they unite, not just in their separate specialties, but as a single professional group. They must increase and widely publicize research that fortifies arguments for quality care and re-commit themselves, their nursing leaders and their nursing educators to confronting conditions that prohibit the full practice of their profession in hospitals. If nurses are willing, not to distance themselves, but to embrace their identity, the revolution is theirs, just as it was for Nightingale years ago.

THE ECONOMIC IMPERATIVE

There is widespread misunderstanding about the high cost of running a hospital. Stories of thirty-dollar aspirins and other hospital items purchased cheaply at the local supermarket have created images of over-pricing and profiteering, while public opinion sometimes overlooks the fact that an elaborate health care delivery network such as a hospital is unique and extremely expensive.

As an institution from which almost every person living and yet unborn will need services, the hospital must not only accommodate individual patients but also be in immediate readiness for events that may require its services at any time without notice. If one considers an institution prepared to provide services to meet any emergency, including disasters that may involve hundreds of people simultaneously in critical need of services, it is incredible to think about how one calculates such costs.

What goes on in a hospital is no less dramatic and requires no less sophisticated resources than those required to land an astronaut on the moon. The activities of an operating room, with the anesthesiologists, surgeons and other highly skilled professionals who must function at their optimum level every moment are crucial to the person on the table. Having five or ten operating theaters running simultaneously is an impressive activity. The physical environment must meet strict specifications. Equipment must not fail, ever. Each doctor, each professional person and each manager in that arena must remain mentally and physically prepared to perform their duties at top level. This is the nature of the legal, fiduciary relationship of the hospital to the community, and it is difficult to put a price on that kind of service.

There is no question that we need wise and innovative business managers to insure the viability of our hospitals. All the passion and energy reserved for commitment to quality care must be accompanied by an equal, if not more aggressive, commitment to the financial integrity of the institution. A facility that does not sustain itself financially through sound fiscal management will cease to exist, and no one benefits. There must also be a surplus, even if the facility is considered non-profit, for the expansion demanded by advancing technology, growing population and changing demography. Furthermore, one must deliver *increasingly* better economic results.

An effective operation of the care delivery process has never been so essential and yet so difficult as it is today. Achieving desired outcomes demands more than mere business management; it demands innovation, creativity and excellence in leadership. It is not merely a matter of cutting costs and raising prices. Nor can we simply discharge the matter by blaming big business or government or allow our energy to be consumed by resistance to inevitable changes in the industry. We must instead focus on taking the direction that will accomplish what we need. If we are to maintain our hospitals, sustain a surplus and deliver increasingly better economic results, we must focus on two things: quality and the creation of new services.

Yet, therein lies the tragedy. Such financial leadership is not happening in many places. Just as the great failure of professionals is their complicity, the great failure of executives is the inability to see that they can only accomplish financial reform, perhaps only survive, in today's health care climate by providing quality care. CEO's often do not realize that many of the staffing patterns, policies and working conditions they design to control the budget only increase the cost of care. Furthermore, they may fail to envision the possibilities in serving the health needs of the community as a whole.

It seems logical to them that early patient discharge should benefit the hospital because most of the revenue is generated during the patient's first few days, particularly for surgical cases. This includes the use of the operating room and other services used early on. The timely discharge of patients *is* important. Yet, many CEO's confuse arbitrary early discharge, pre-determined by guidelines, with quality and healing. Eventually, the accumulated consequences of such poor insight, that is, costly patient complications and re-admissions, are devastating to the financial goals of the hospital.

It seems logical to many CEO's that decreasing professional service will decrease the cost of running the institution. They do not take into account any other result. All the while, expensive lawsuits, patient complications, increased lengths of stay, and re-admissions rise. Both professional and non-professional employee turnover also rises.

Many CEO's fail to grasp the fact that the hospital's product is *service*. It is the most important factor that differentiates one facility from another, either attracting or repelling both patients and professionals. Offering better or more service automatically means more money for the bottom line. The nursing staff, the largest number of professionals qualified to produce the hospital's product are not best categorized as a cost center, but a *revenue center.*

One of the greatest afflictions of some of our hospitals is management from the top-level by intimidation, which naturally compels many CEO's to practice job safety, to avoid risk-taking so vital to success, failing to determine what are appropriate, even essential, risks and what are not.

Consequently, they themselves do not encourage, indeed they create no opportunities for, nurses and other caregivers to experiment and to demonstrate better methods with greater economic returns.

The courage to remain truly focused on the hospital's mission and to act on principle can be very difficult to muster. Fortunately, there are those for whom the awareness of opportunities, resources and power to produce change are so invigorating that the obstacles are welcome challenges. Yet, even for those who begin to experience success, it is still difficult to *stay the course* in the face of skepticism and criticism encountered when advancing ideas outside the norm. This can remain true even as many of the skeptics and the critics themselves accept some of the ideas and began to use them.

Amid these and any number of other such obstacles, CEO's must then turn their attention to their day job, that is, the leadership of others, creating an environment in which those persons can render their best work. In the end, the ability, or lack thereof, of the CEO to provide the environment in which professionals can perform at their highest level is where the CEO's credit or discredit lies. This is the dynamic that determines the ultimate economic success or failure of the hospital.

To be successful, the CEO's must first see that managers understand their product. Since the business is about healing, the objective is to be *better* at it, to accelerate it. And if managers are to enable persons at the bedside to provide excellent professional service, to accelerate the healing of patients, then they must be committed to the critical care the caregivers themselves need. The employees must be expected to act in any situation for the safety and well being of patients and other employees, according to a set of guidelines that empowers them. Managers must perpetually empower caregivers to innovate. They must enable and expect the people delivering direct care to improve and design systems they deem worthwhile and to study the results, including bottom line.

Managers must work as a team, not necessarily in agreement, but always as a team, thinking not only of their independent positions but also of the broader responsibility of the CEO. They must be the authors, discoverers and implementers of ideas. Even the managers of small community hospitals must assume their service can be as good as, or better than, that of anyone in the country. They too must make a case for their objectives and tell the CEO what they need. Strong communication between bedside caregivers and managers, between managers and CEO's, also results in fewer unresolved problems, leaving more energy for innovation. Some hospitals facilitate this through advisory councils, but it should also be accomplished through day to day freedom to express ideas and opinions. The difference such an approach makes in any facility is palpable, and the outcome of such dynamics is economic success.

Economic success can also result from the expanding of services. Successful CEO's extend their responsibility beyond merely managing the hospital to preserving the quality of life and health in the community. They are convinced of the absolute importance of their institution to the community, viewing the hospital as a manufacturing plant for services. As advocates for the health of the community, they may find ways to aid in community emergency preparedness, public health education, emergency medical service training, child abuse prevention and an infinite number of other services. When the captain of a local fire department suffered a heart attack, one CEO offered a heart attack prevention program to the firemen.

During a hepatitis epidemic, the CEO contacted the health department director and simply asked, "What can we do to help?"

As it happened, the health department director was sending lab work out of town and waiting a considerable length of time for results. The hospital acquired the fairly inexpensive means of offering the laboratory service faster at the hospital, for which the health department director was grateful, and the hospital benefited from the additional revenue.

If nursing home patients came into the hospital, and it was evident that they had not received good care prior to their coming, the hospital notified the appropriate agencies. Three substandard nursing homes in the community were closed as a result of the hospital's efforts.

People who run hospitals or have influence over the model of care that is provided must recognize that they are social architects in constantly changing communities. They can actively engage in designing the future of health care in their community. There are no real constraints on what they can offer. If they do not drift away from their commitment to quality care and their fiduciary relationship to the community, if they view that commitment as absolute, they will create and invest in needed services both within the hospital and within the community as a whole.

Obviously, one's hospital-running education does not end with a university diploma; it begins with the job. The university inculcates the importance of a profitable bottom line, but it cannot possibly teach future CEO's all the ways to get there, and it may not distinguish those methods that are most compatible with quality and service. Furthermore, there is a certain amount of bungy jumping involved, which is also neglected in the university education.

One CEO recounts an incident that illustrates this point:

"I was out of the hospital one afternoon when the regional director called. Since I was not in, he spoke directly to the person who lists laboratory prices, instructing her to increase all charges by ten percent. When I returned, she informed me that she had done so. My first response was to remind her respectfully that she did not work for the regional director; she worked for me. I then told her to remove all the charges, that I was sorry to ask her to do the extra work, but there would be no increase in lab charges."

"She said, 'What are you going to do?'"

"I said, 'I'll figure it out before tomorrow.'"

"The problem was that the regional director had recently addressed the medical staff and told them that there would be no more increases that year. Now, three weeks later, he called, because corporate called him, telling us to increase the charges. (He had been CEO at our facility before I was, and he was still running the hospital from the regional office, he thought.) But our lab charges were already high. A new blood chemistry test in particular was the most expensive charge, and for that reason, the doctors weren't using it, even though it would benefit their patients."

"The next morning I called him and said, 'I wanted to let you know that I got your message about the lab charges. I have to ask you to trust that I know what I'm doing, but I'm not increasing the charges, and here's why: You were up here three weeks ago...' and I went through what he'd said then. I added, 'Do you realize you will have no respect from our doctors if you go against your word? I don't want that to happen.'"

"I then sent memos to the doctors explaining that I knew they weren't using the new test, even when they would like to, because the charge was so high. I understood where they were coming from, and I wanted them to know that the cost of the test had been reduced twenty-five percent."

"The doctors began ordering it at twice the rate of before. My laboratory revenue for the month was higher than all my charges. It exceeded what I was expected to do. The patients benefited; the doctors were pleased, and the corporation couldn't believe it."

This small example of increasing revenue while decreasing prices was appropriate risk-taking because it was driven by values placing the patient's needs first. CEO's must be very clear on what is right, what is required for patients. Such clarity provides built-in courage and daring.

Another means of increasing bottom line is one that is viewed with trepidation by many CEO's, but a lay-off, if necessary and if handled well, is not a sin. Sometimes, it is better for everyone around. But the criterion for determining who will be included in the lay-off has to be poor work, not length of employment or salary. Department managers, having been informed of the number of persons they are to let go, choose those persons, explain to them why, and *assist them* with filing unemployment insurance and finding other employment.

Admittedly, it is a process that should be closely monitored because it can go badly if not carried out in the best way. But when this logical and humane approach is taken, a lay-off does not demoralize or create anxiety among the other employees; it instead raises morale. And it allows for better ways to spend the money.

The competitive edge will be achieved by very few in the hospital industry. Those few will be extremely successful, and their success will be determined by several critical factors: They will have courage. They will ask the right questions. They will recognize positive change, embrace it and be excited by it. They will harness the energy of their most fragile and critical resources, their human resources, and create working conditions that will cause people to want to come to work for them rather than their competition. They will have at the bedside those individuals who take seriously their responsibility to participate in creating the necessary systems to accomplish accelerated healing. And when student professionals come for training at their facility, they may well see a higher, not lower, standard than they are being taught in the classroom.

To be successful in the hospital industry begins with understanding one's mission and being able to convey, both to patients and caregivers, that one has such understanding. It means working everyday to meet the simple but formidable challenge to remain centered on the patient and the community, reminding one's self daily, even hourly, of the hospital's purpose. And it means consistently incorporating that mindset into the task at hand everyday.

Today's CEO's must search out *simplicity*. A complex solution to a complex problem is not a good solution. Amid an infinite variety of buzzwords and convoluted deal-making, one must remain focused on the hospital's simple mission. To lose sight of the elegance of simplicity, the simple responsibility for serving each other and the dignity of work is to be at the dying edge.

Simple is by no means necessarily easy. Each leader in today's health industry must look into their organizations and find that small but crucial group of persons with a little courage. They are the persons with whom you will build the best health care facility at the best cost.

0-595-21883-0

51333712R00095

Made in the USA
Lexington, KY
20 April 2016